List of Flowers

African violet
Alstroemeria
Anemone

Begonia
Buttercup

Calla Liliy
Camellia
Canna
Carnation
Chrysanthemum
Clematis
Columbine
Cornflower
Crocus
Cyclamen

Daffodil
Dahlia
Daisy

Freesia

Gardenia
Geranium
Gerbera Daisy
Gladiolus

Hibiscus
Hyacinth
Hydrangea

Iris

Lavender
Lily

Magnolia

Orchid

Peony
Petunia
Phlox
Poppy

Rose

Sunflower
Sweet Pea

Tea rose
Transvaal daisy
Tulip

Zinnia

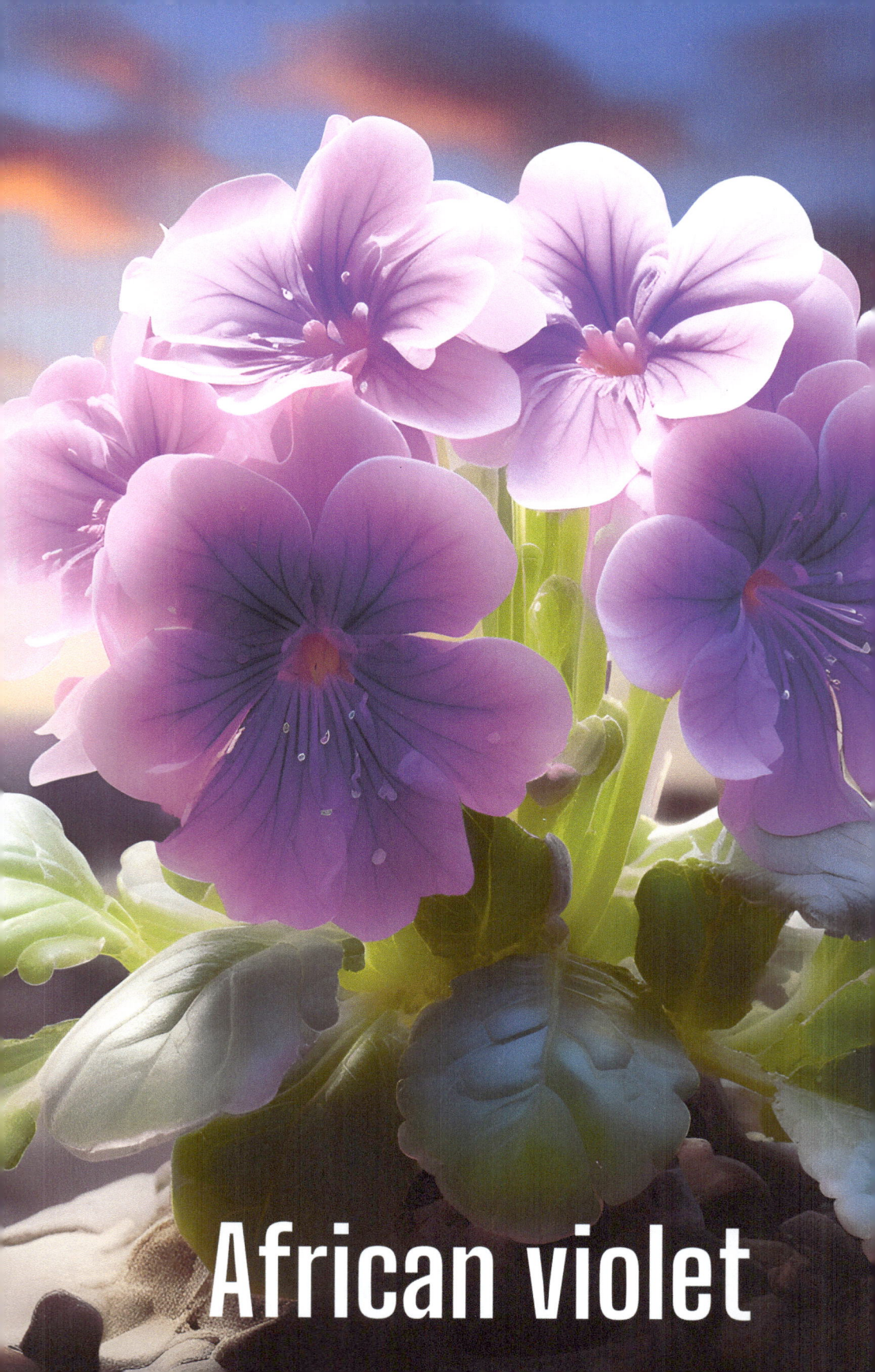

African violet

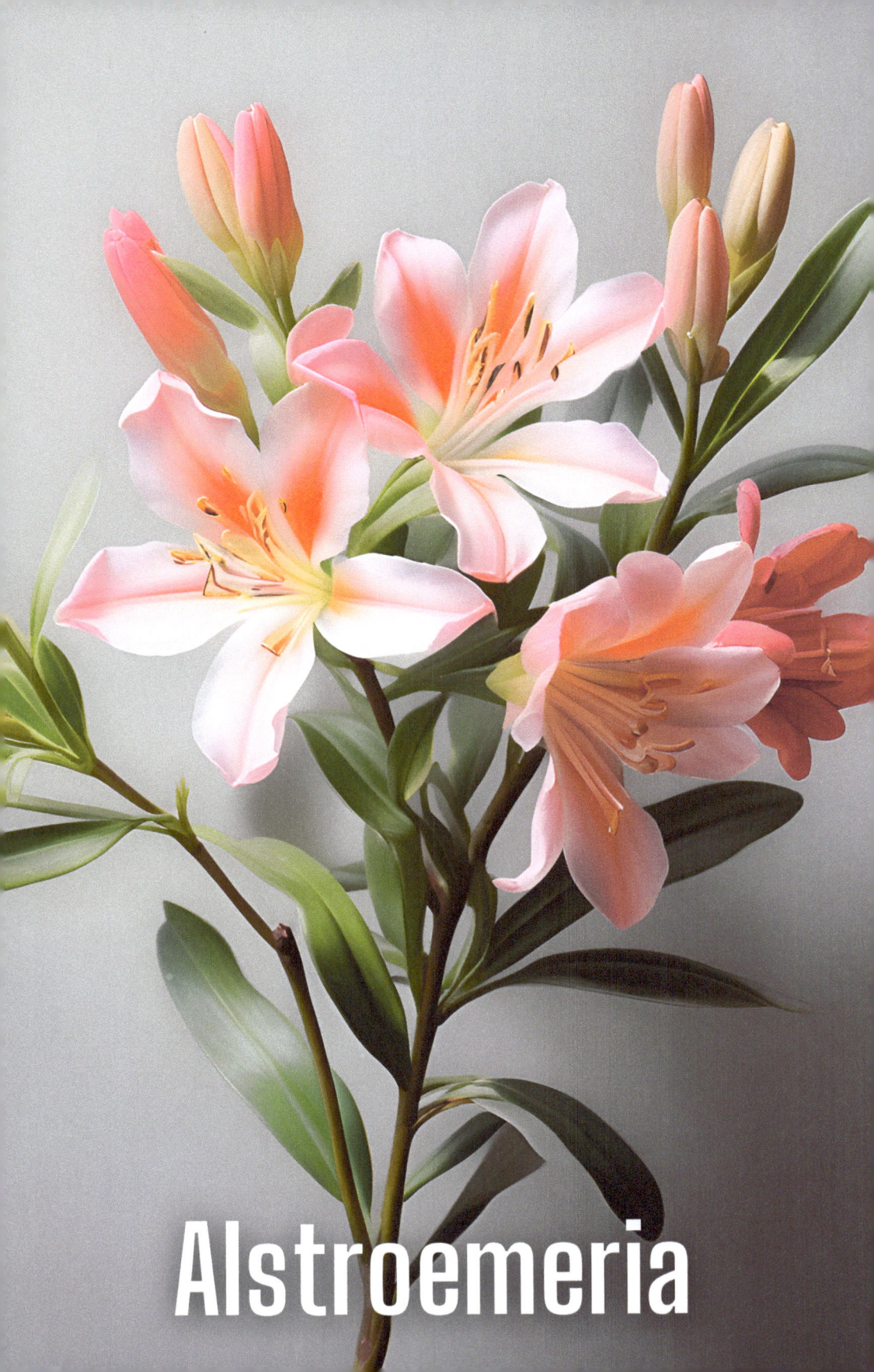

Alstroemeria

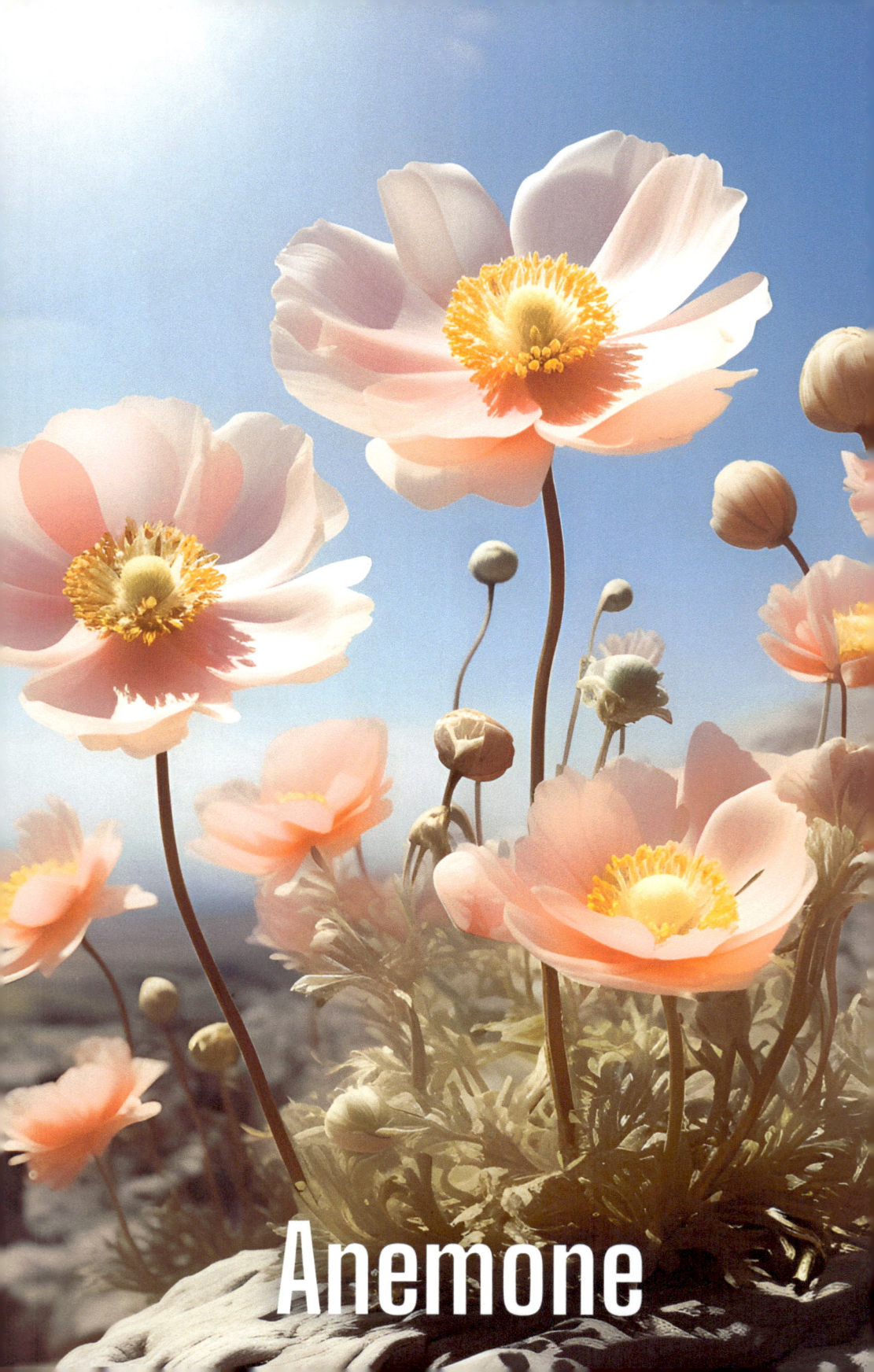

Anemone

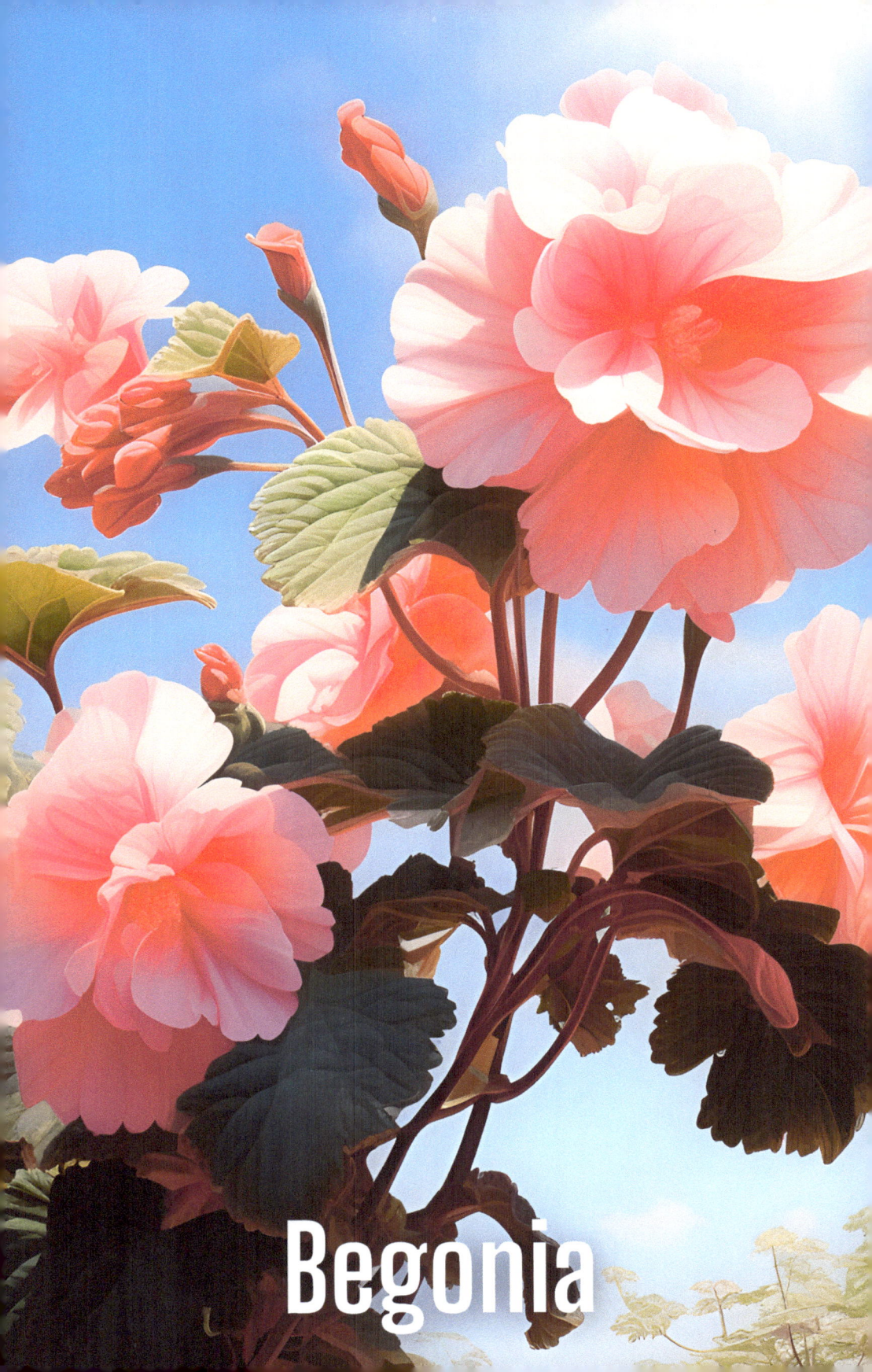

Begonia

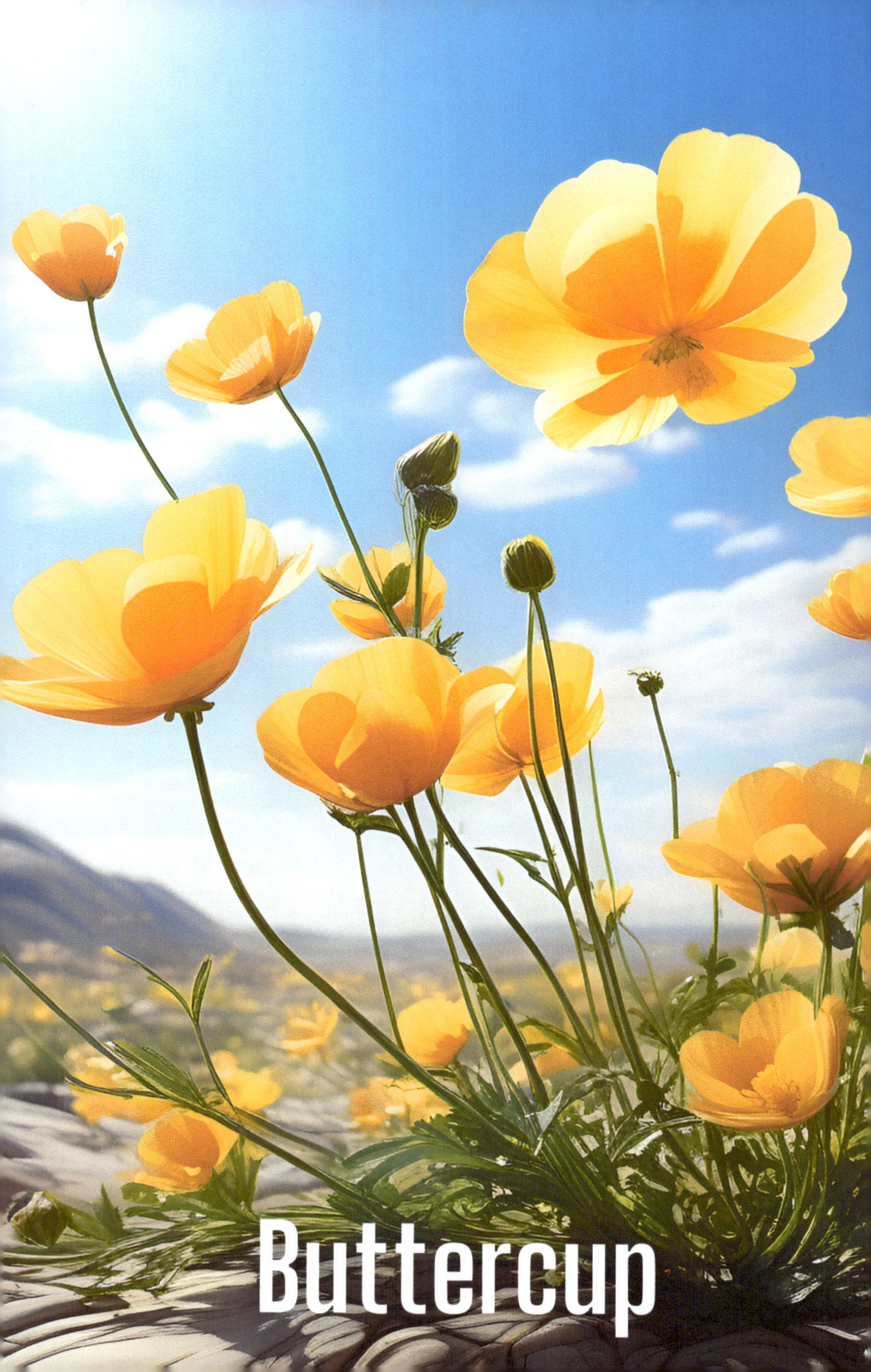

Buttercup

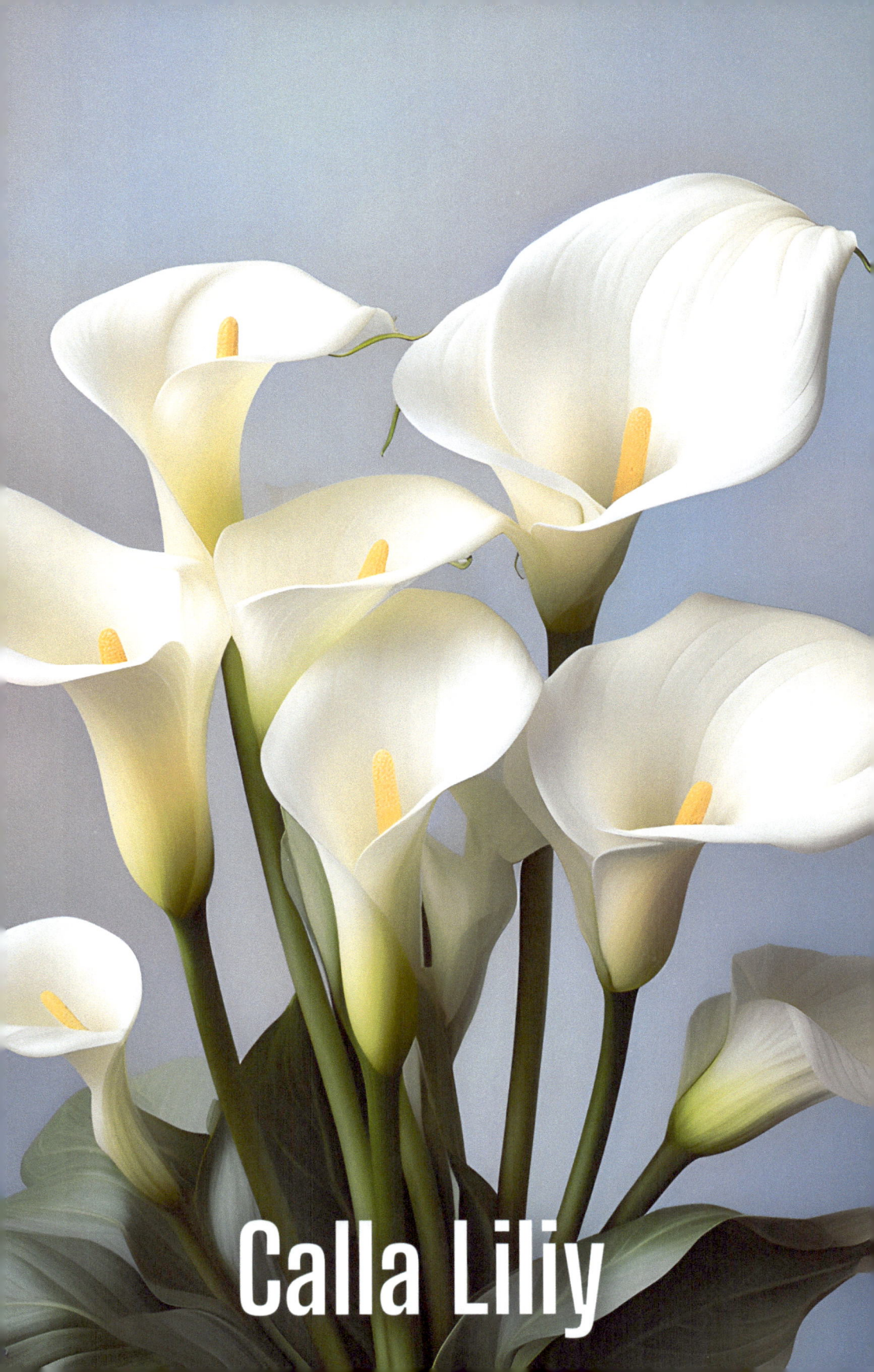

Calla Liliy

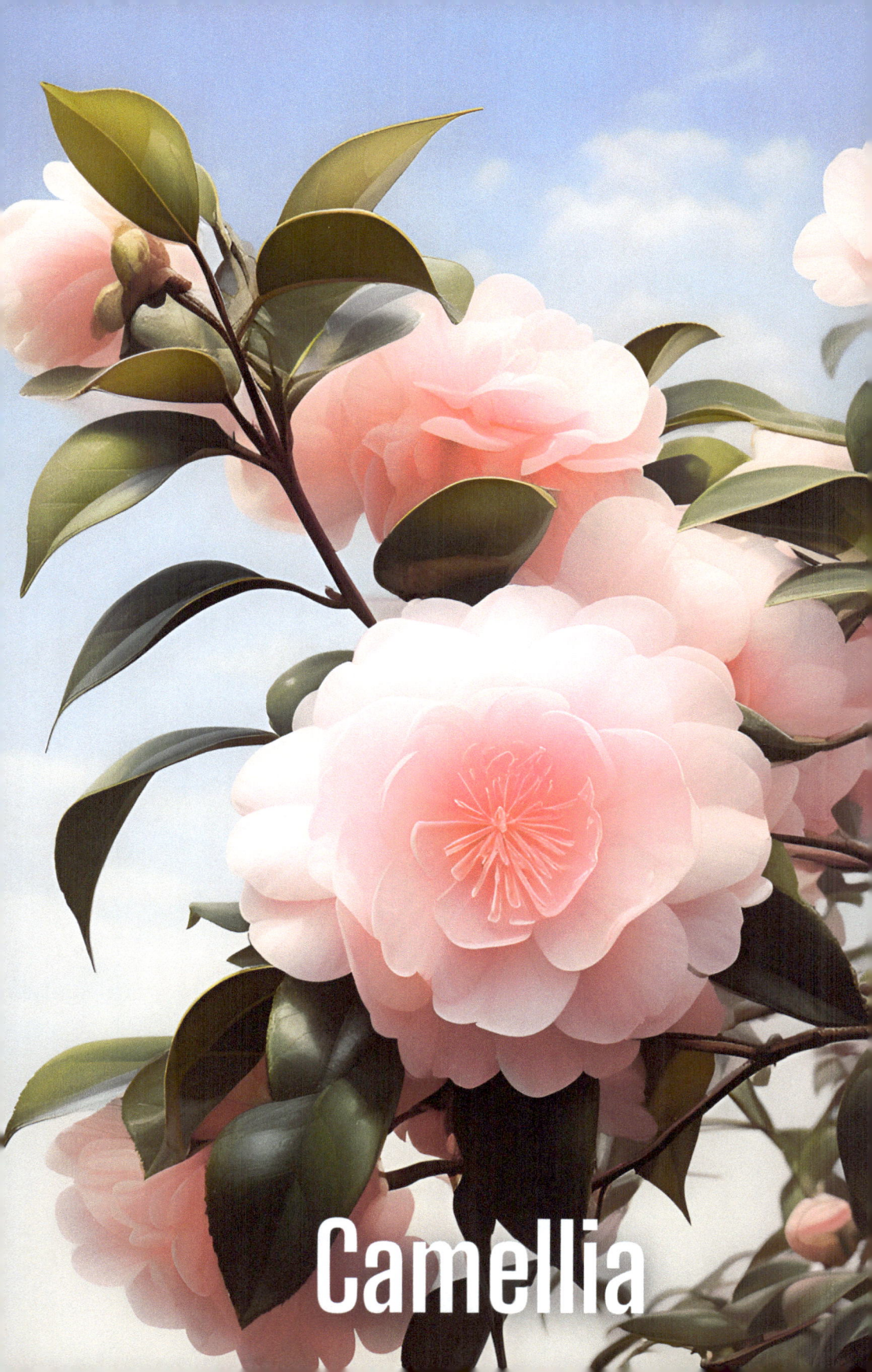

Camellia

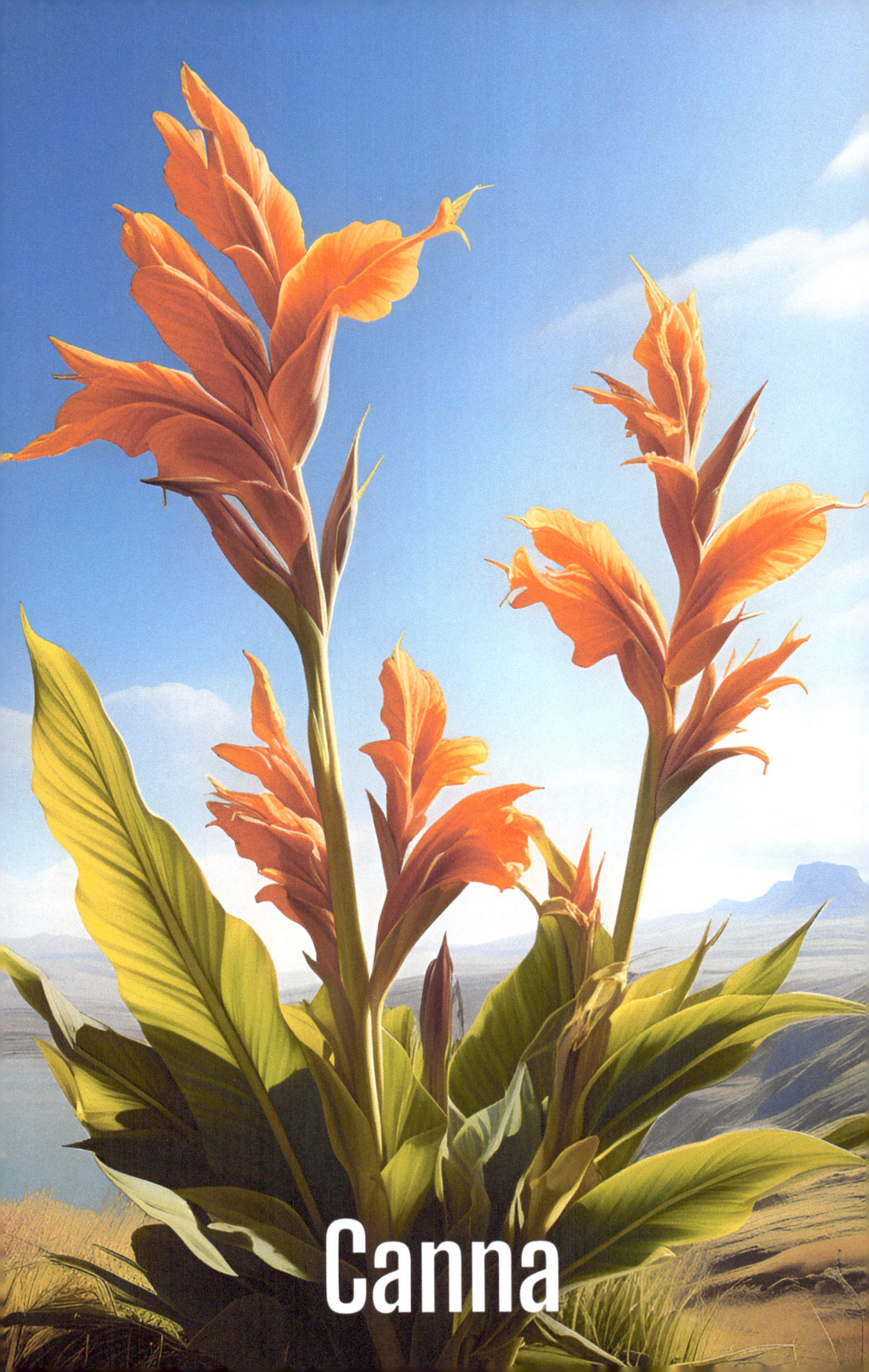

Canna

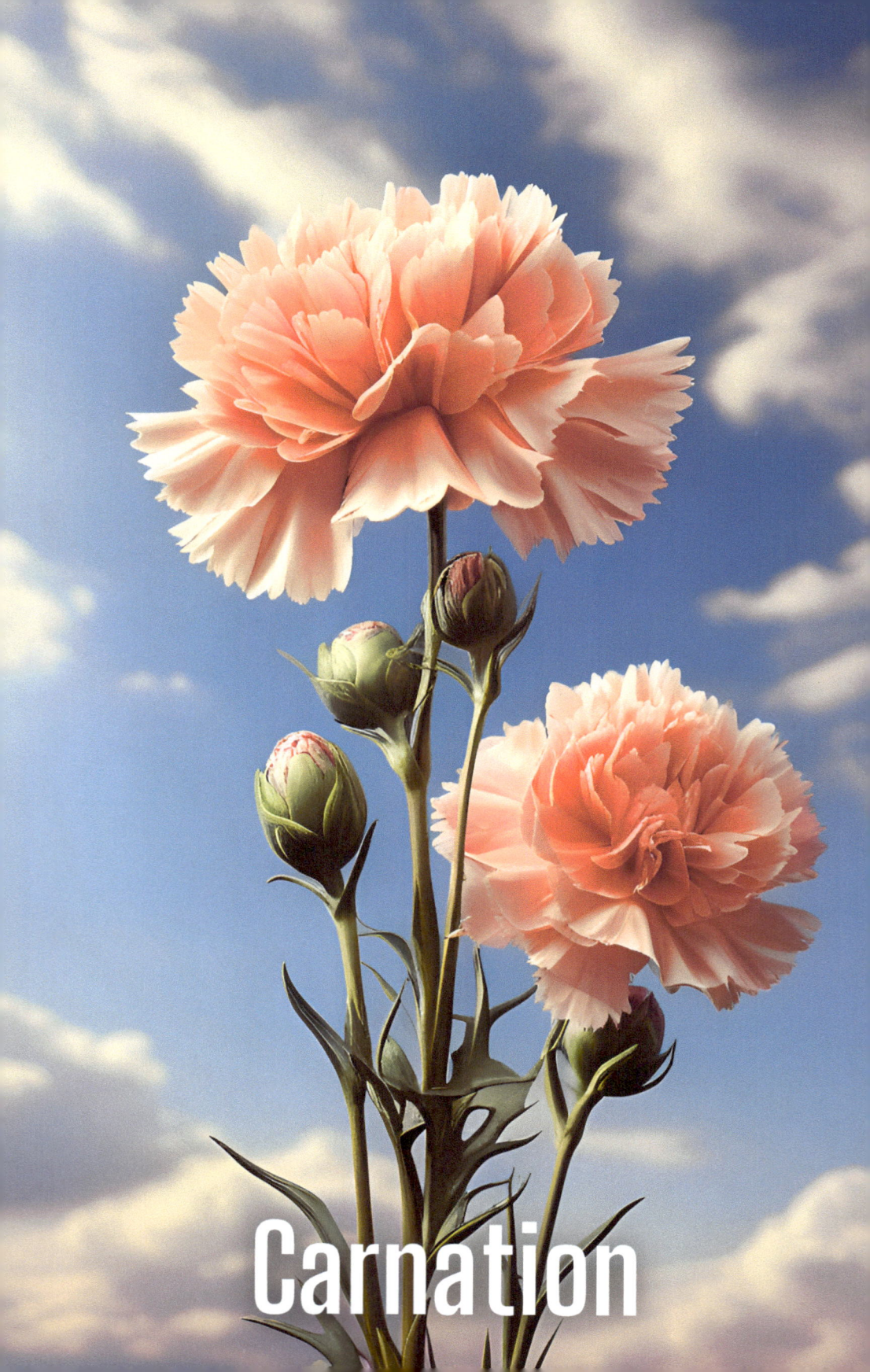

Carnation

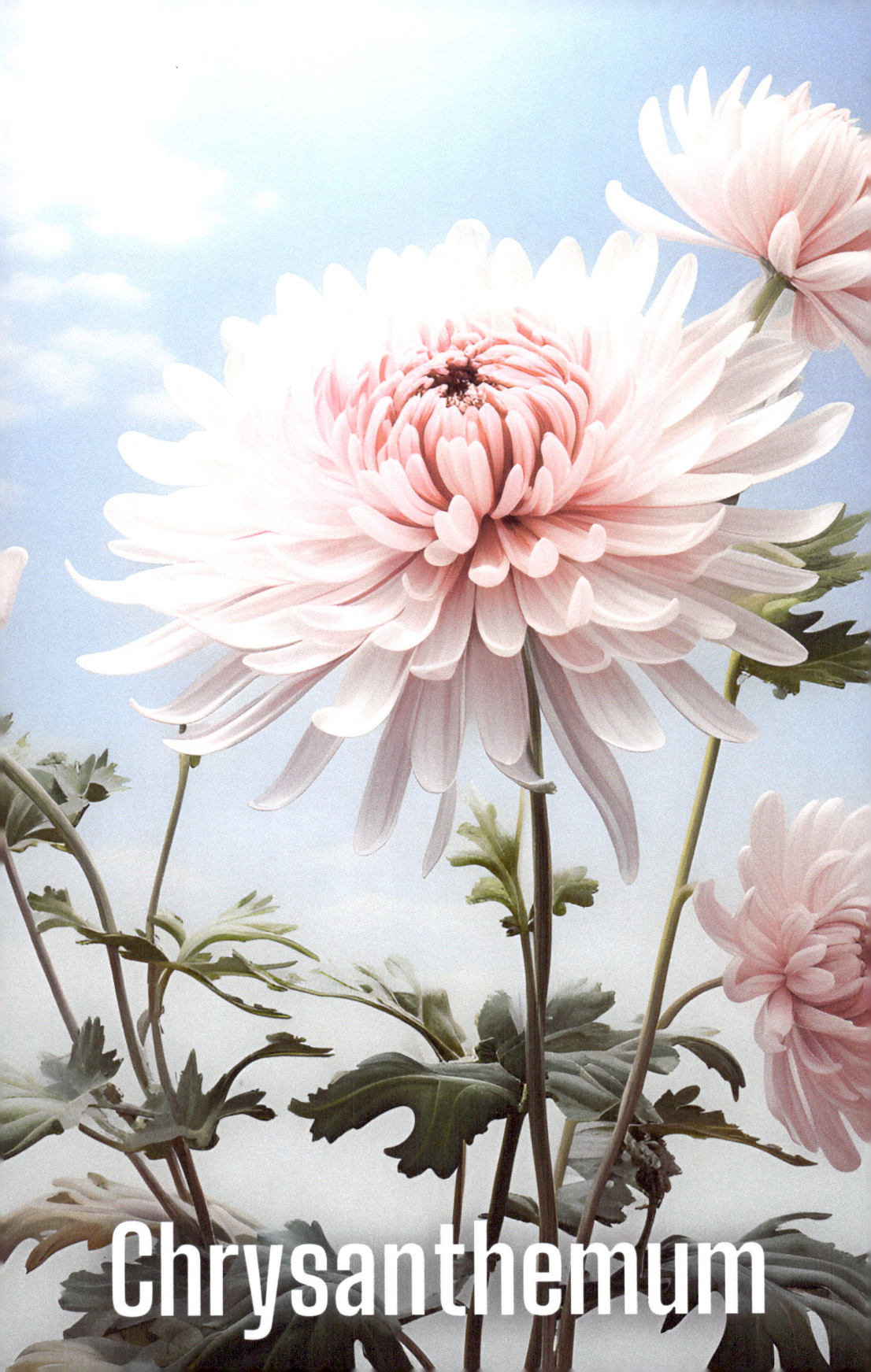

Chrysanthemum

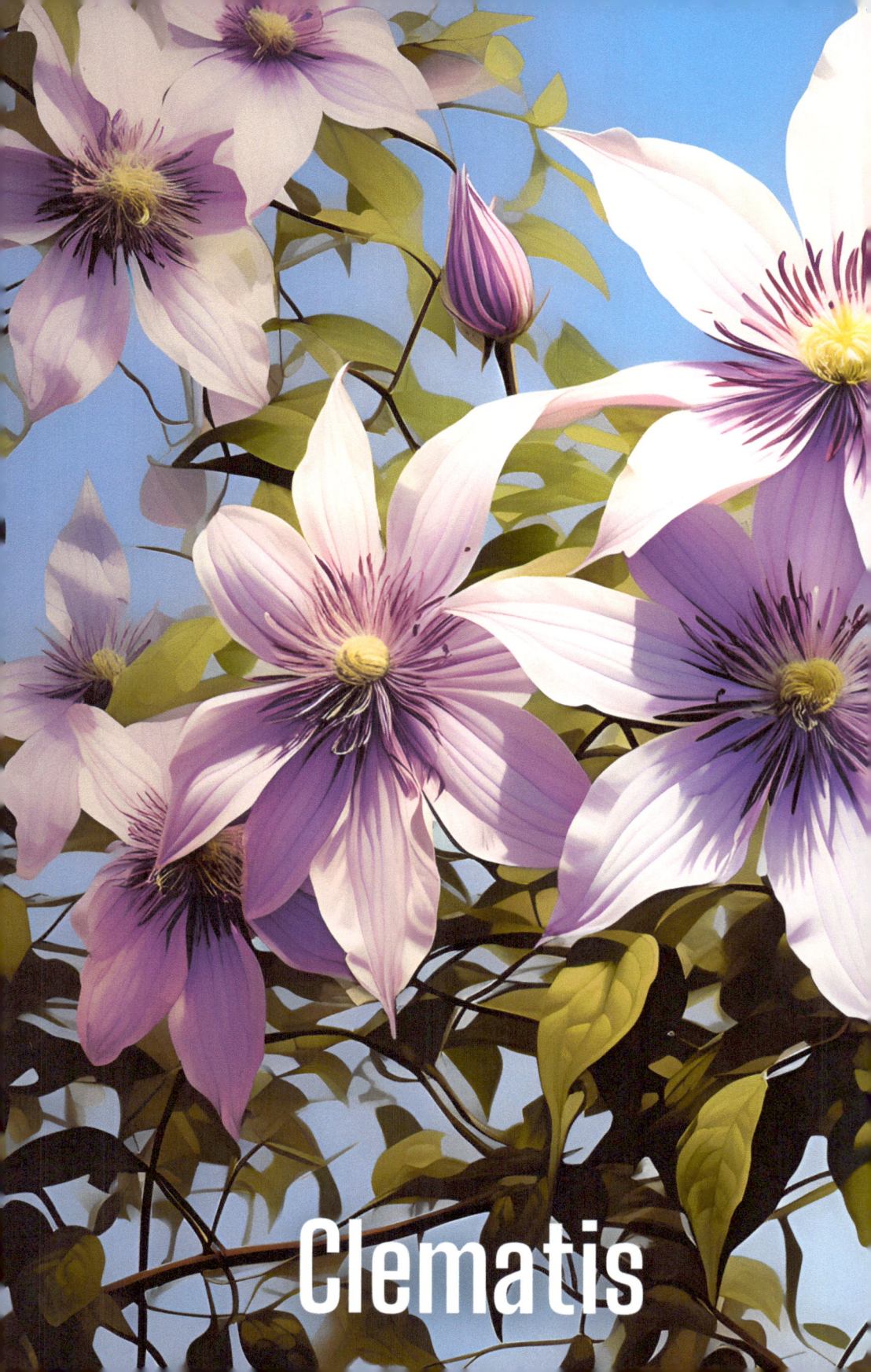

Clematis

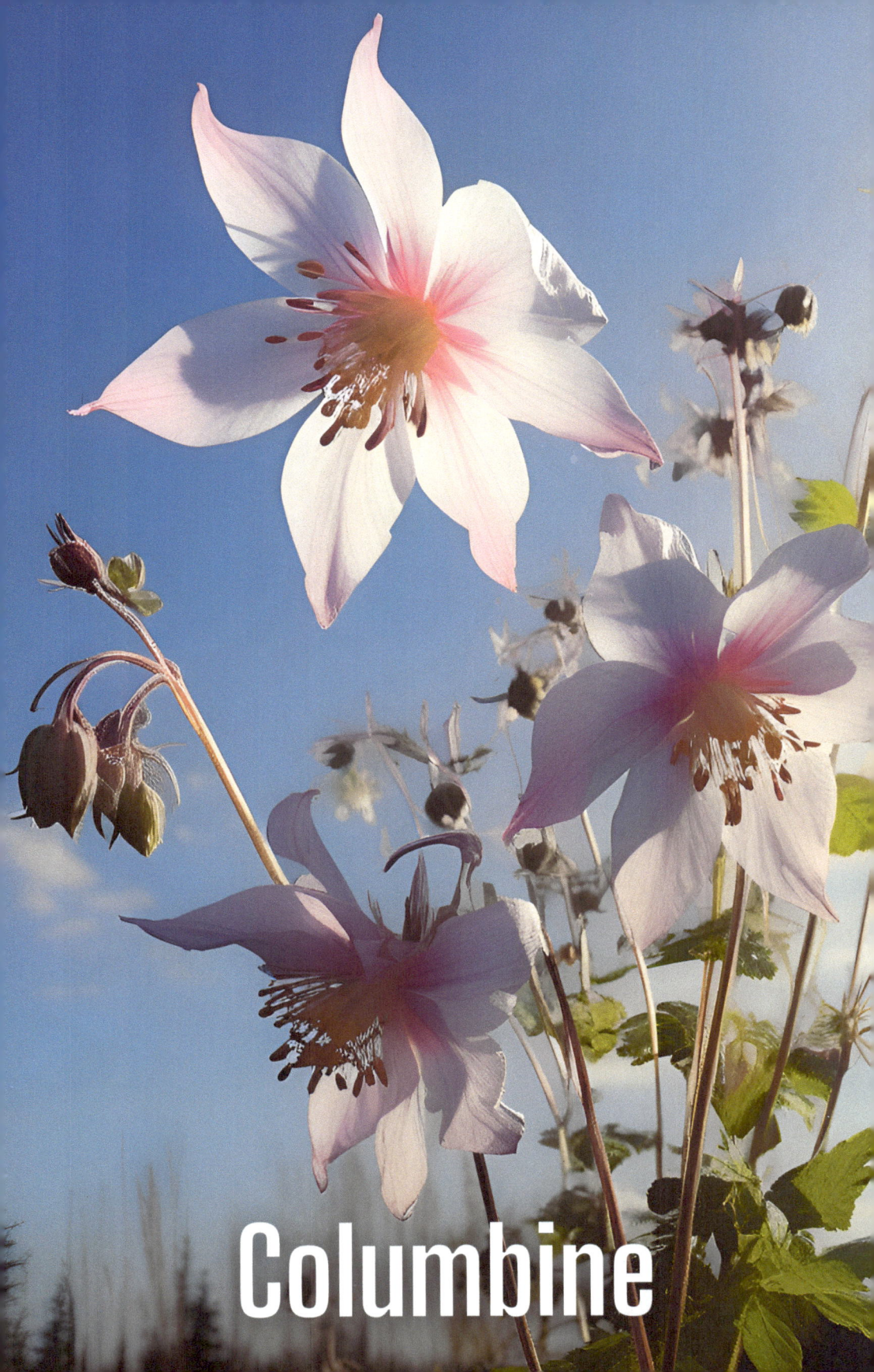

Columbine

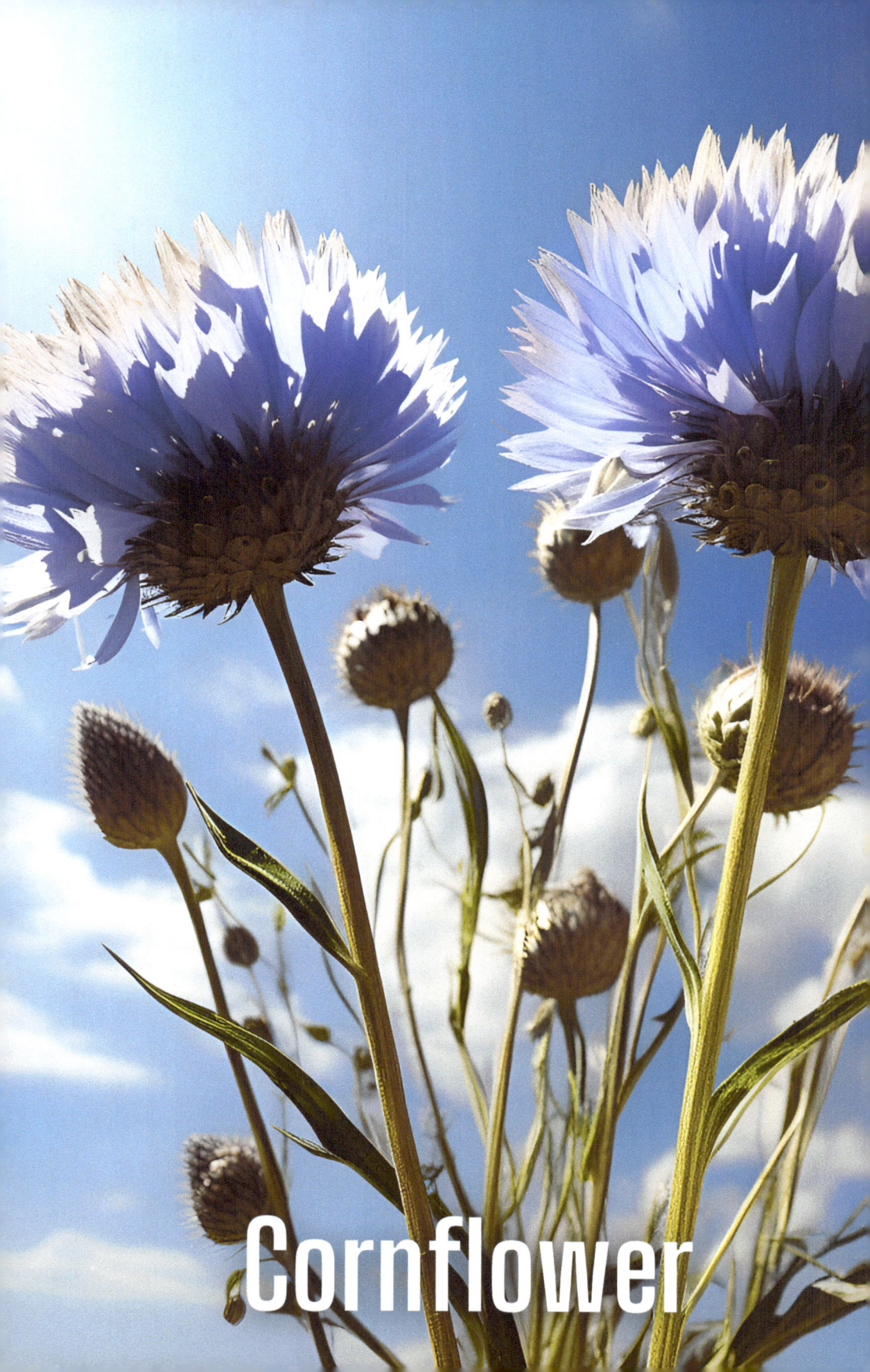

Cornflower

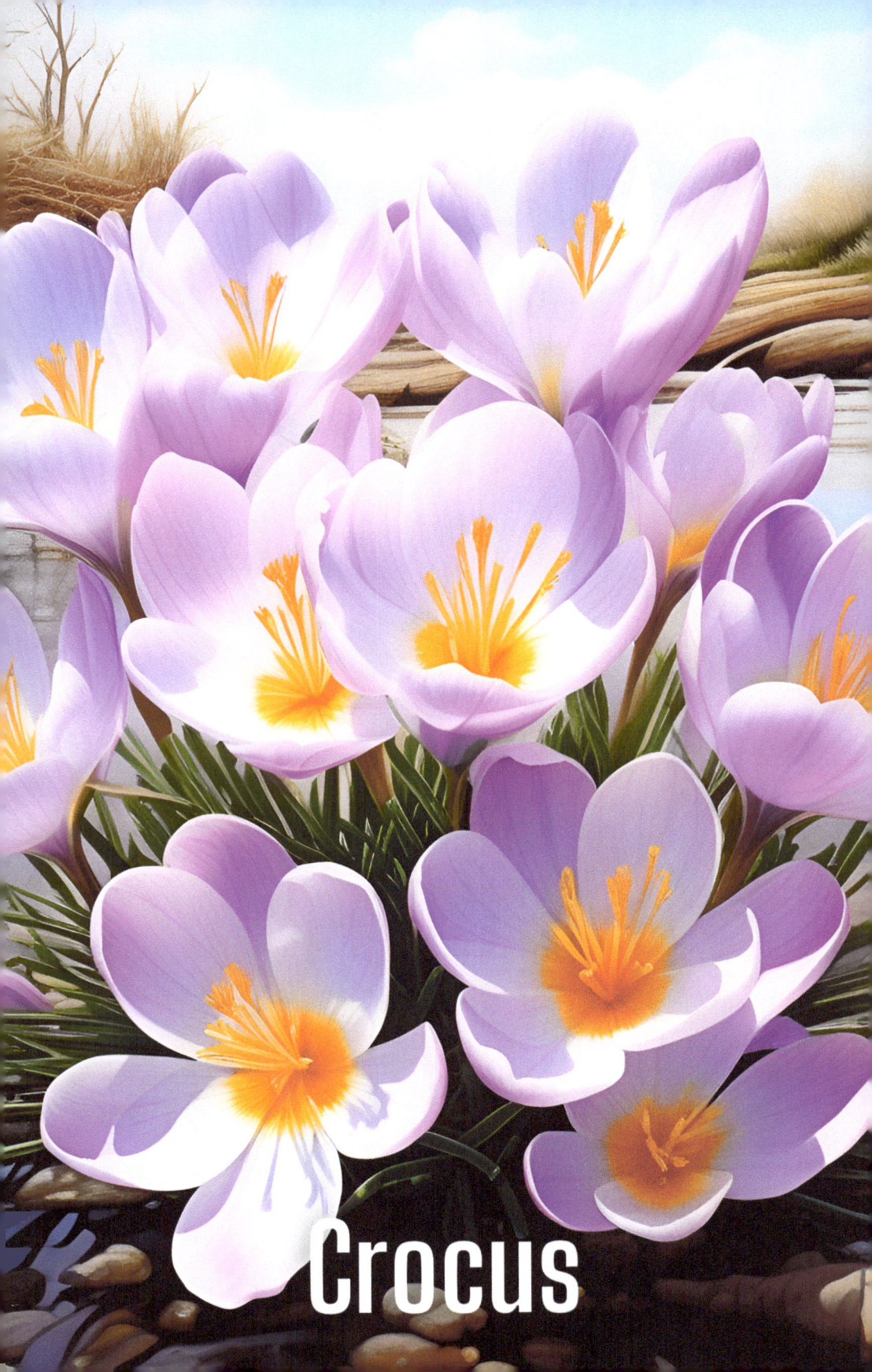

Crocus

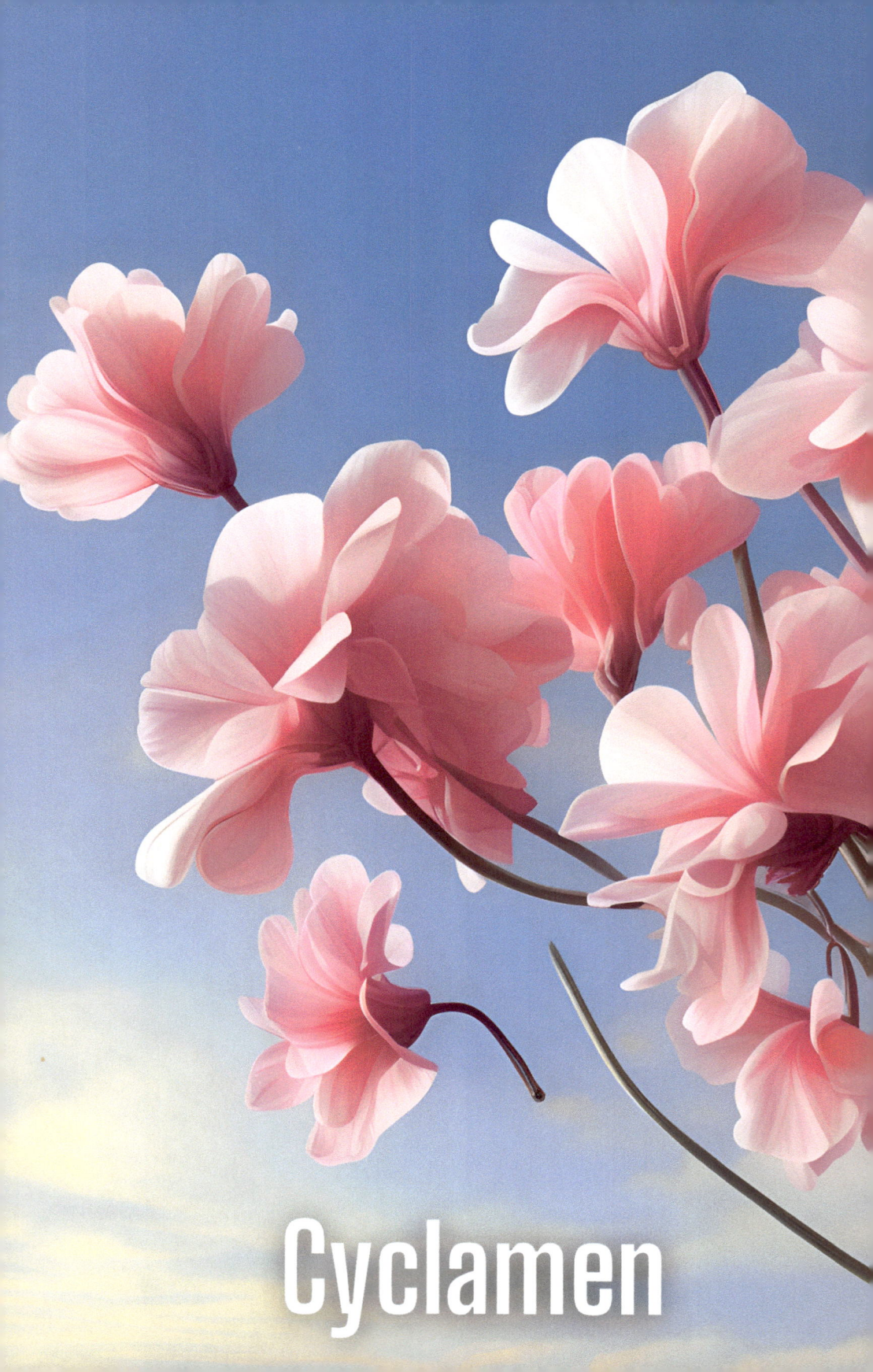

Cyclamen

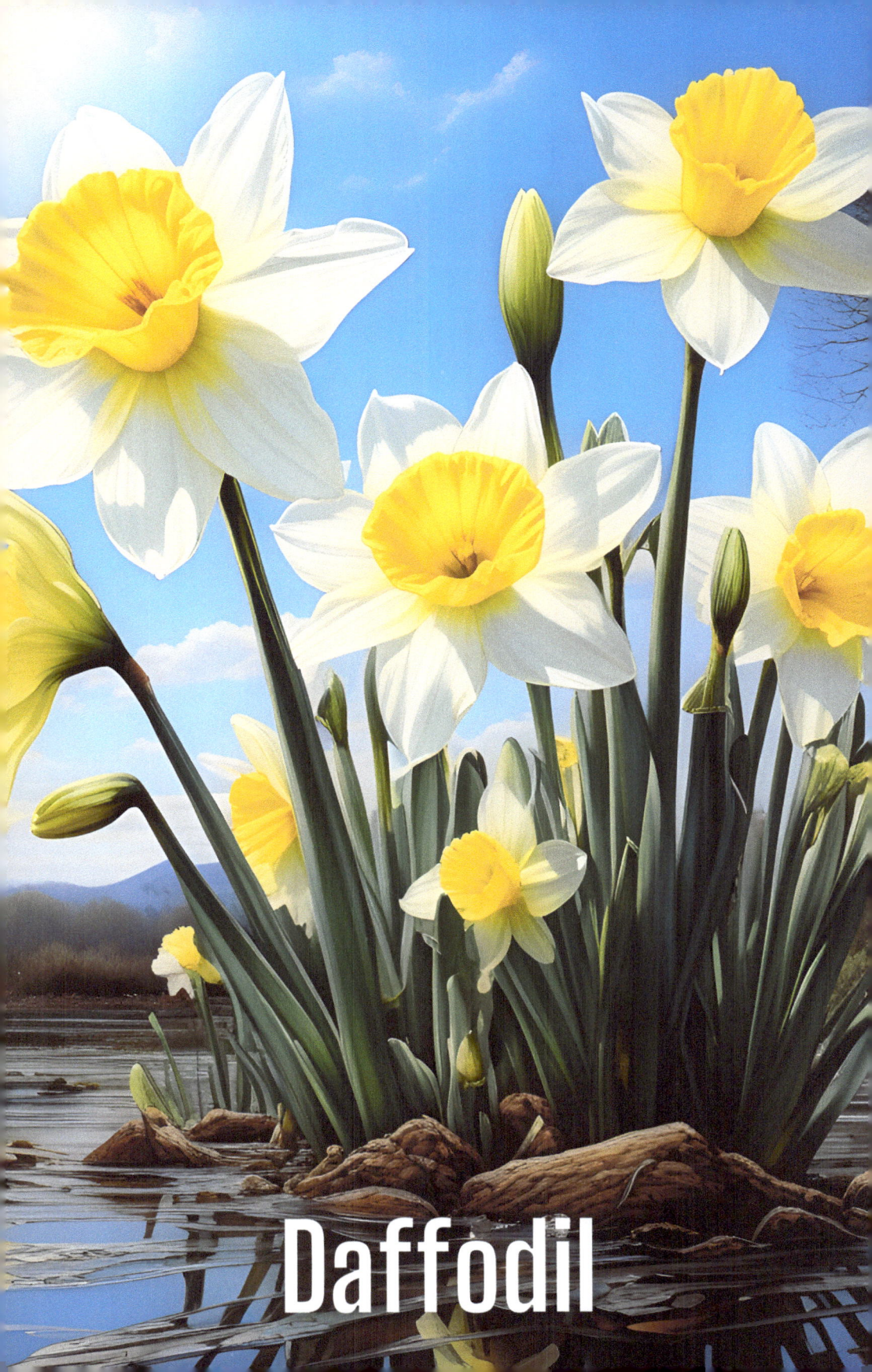

Daffodil

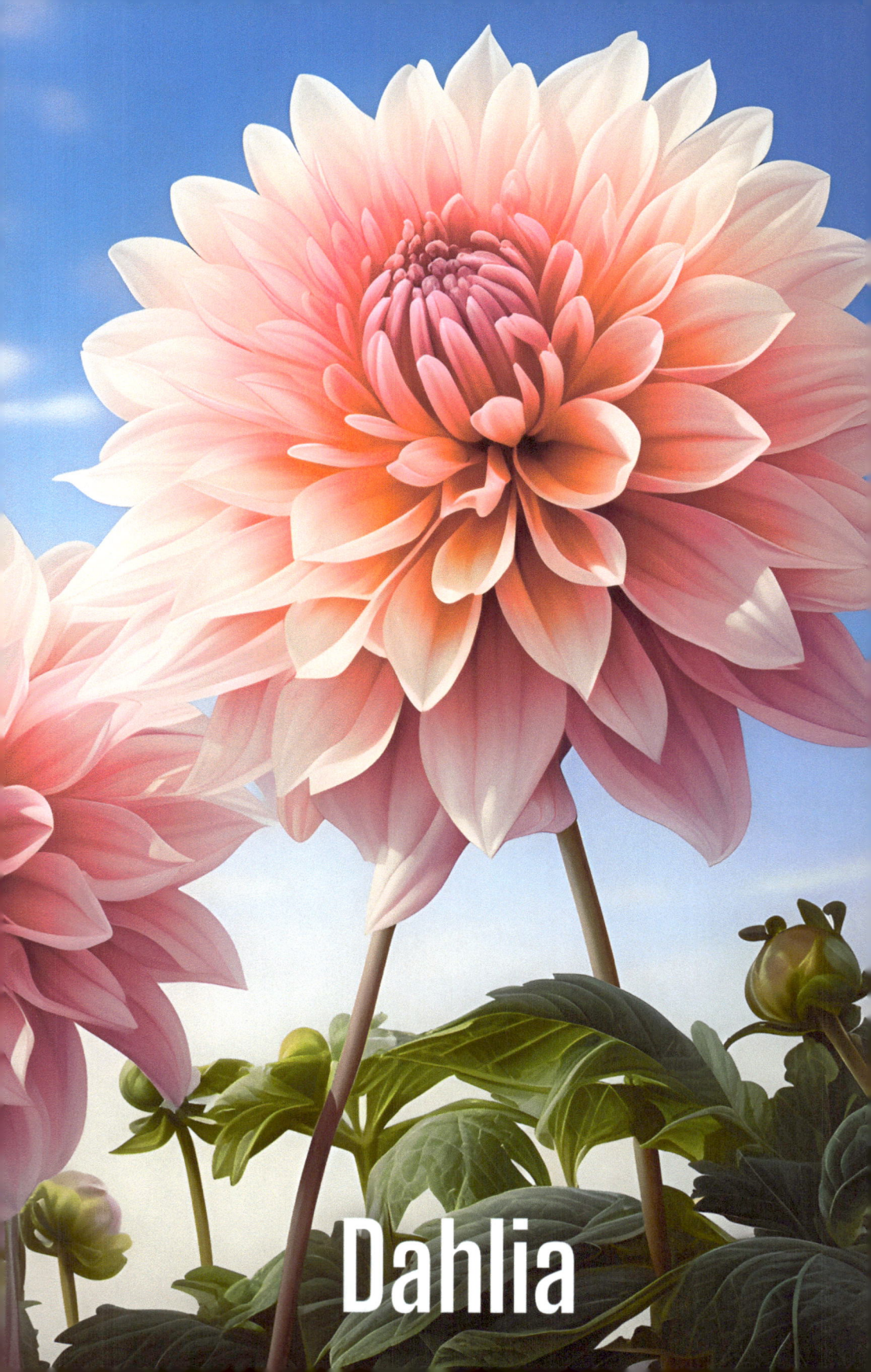

Dahlia

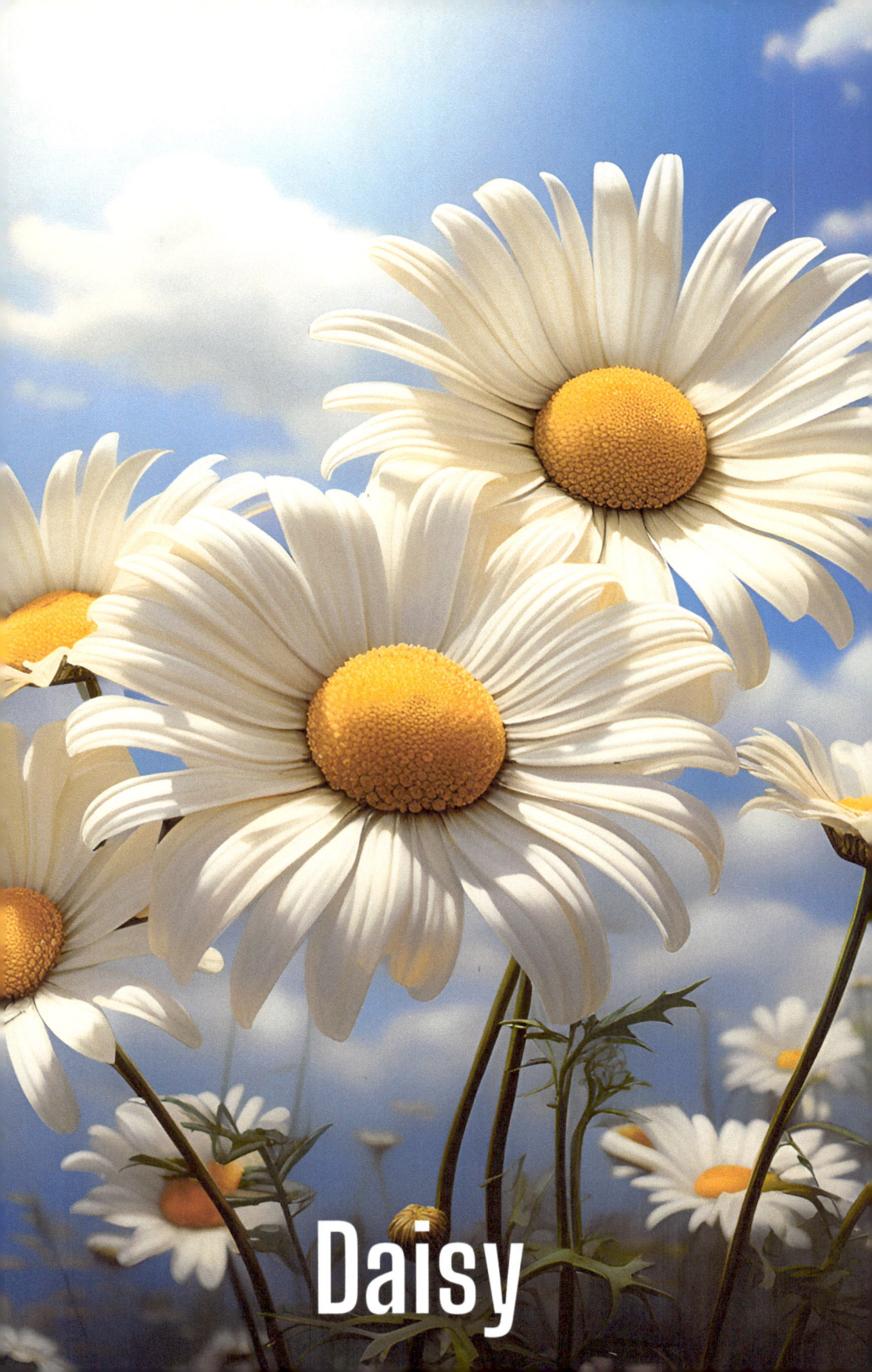

Daisy

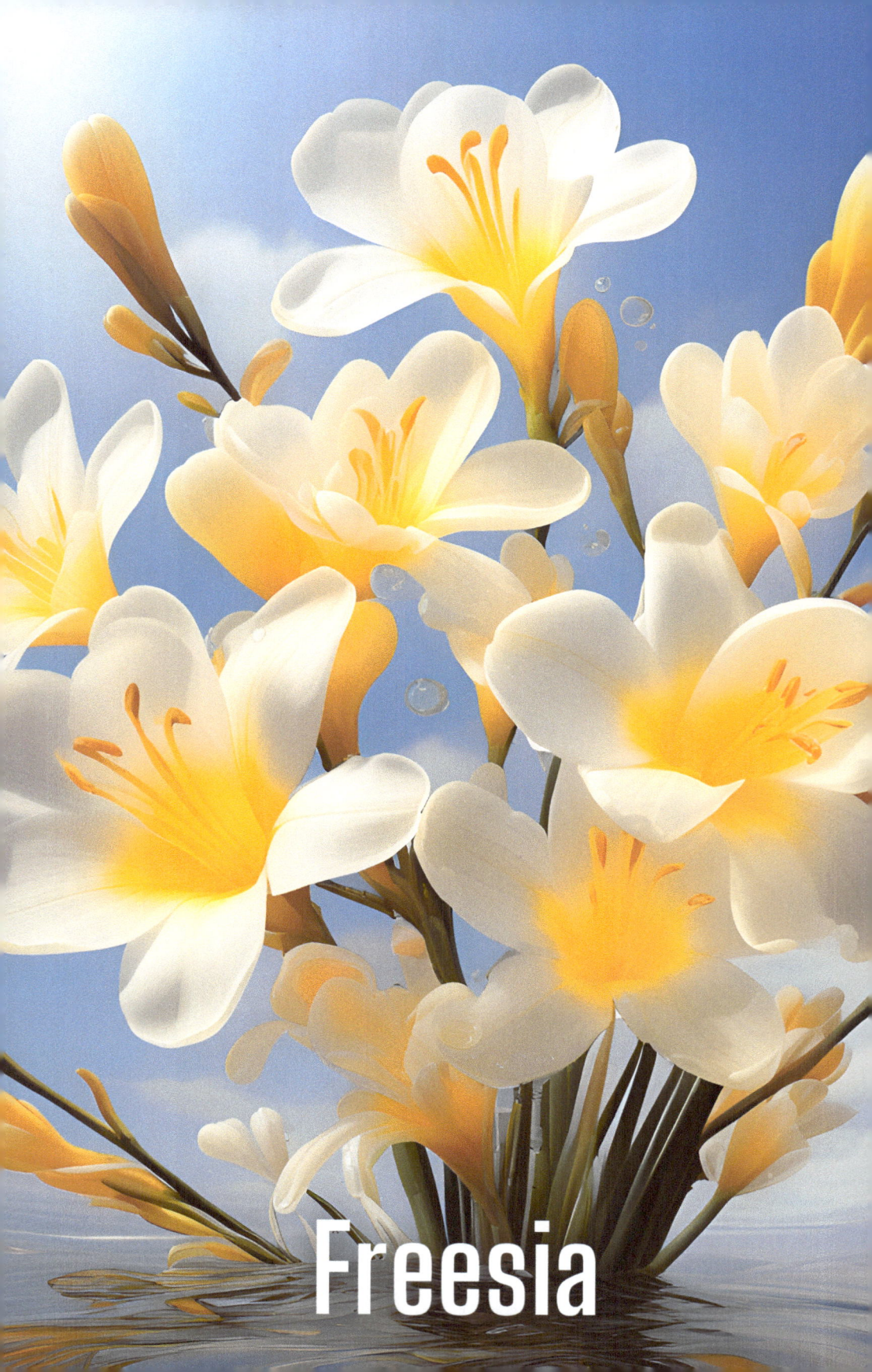

Freesia

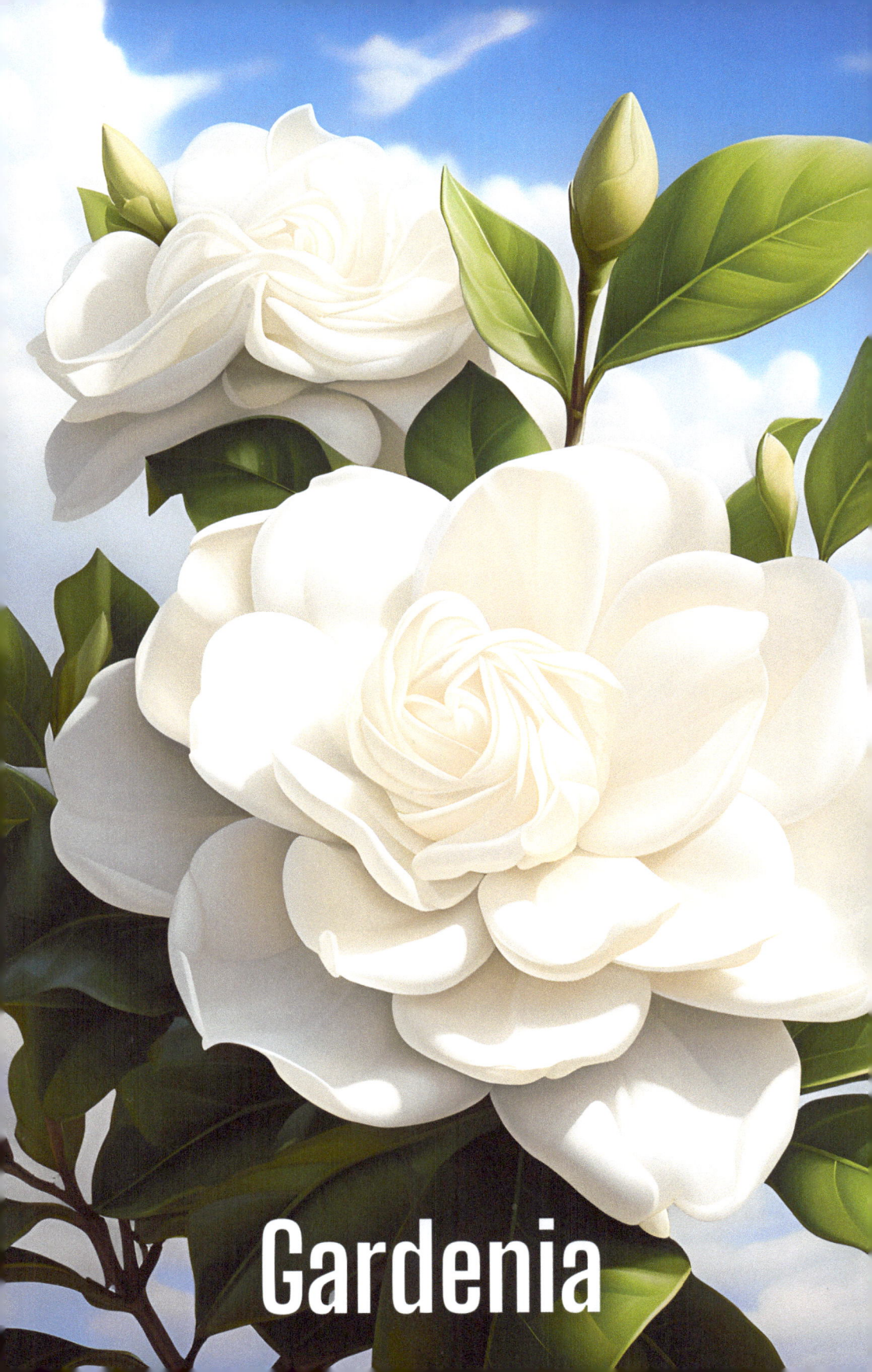

Gardenia

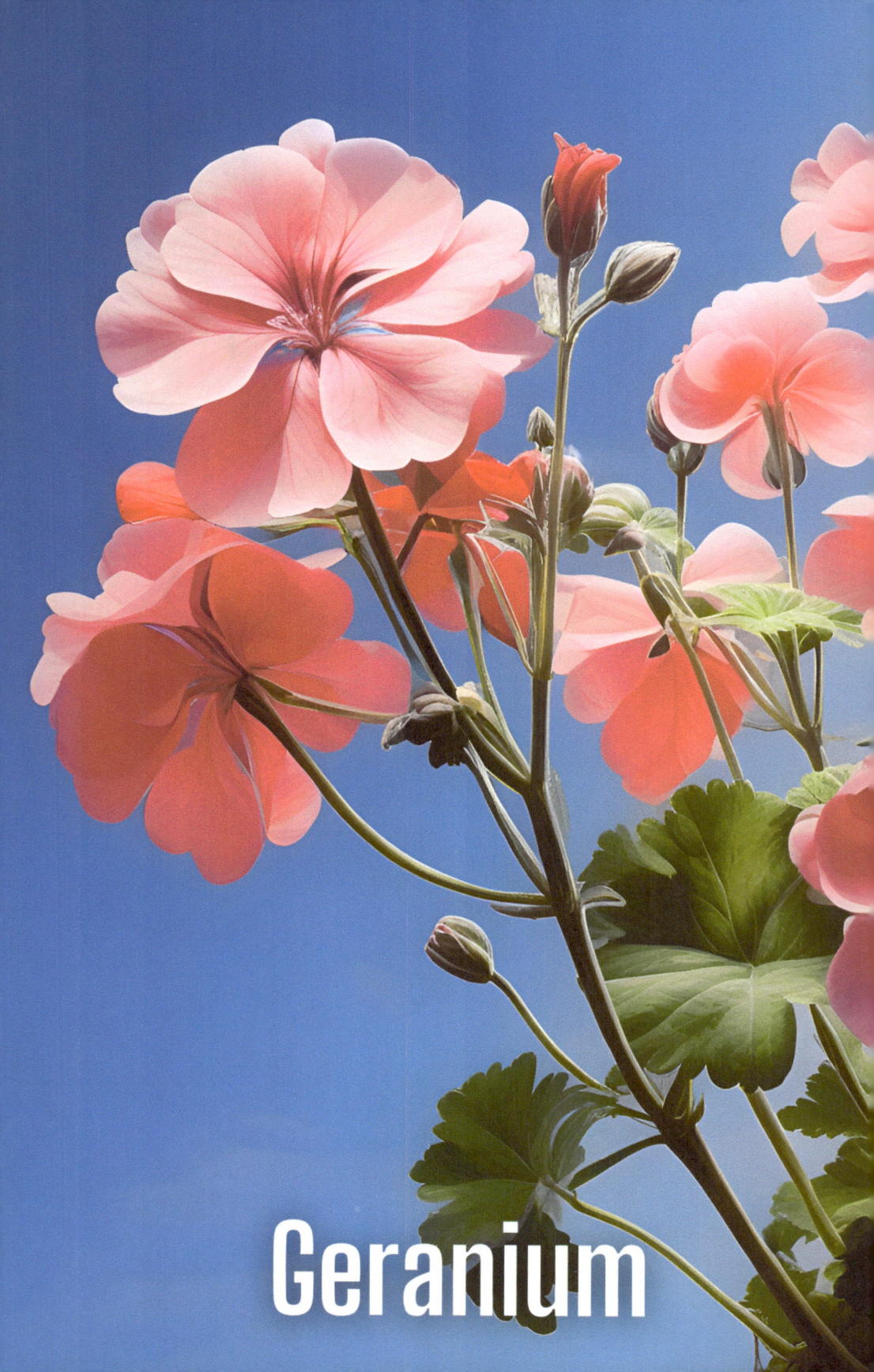

Geranium

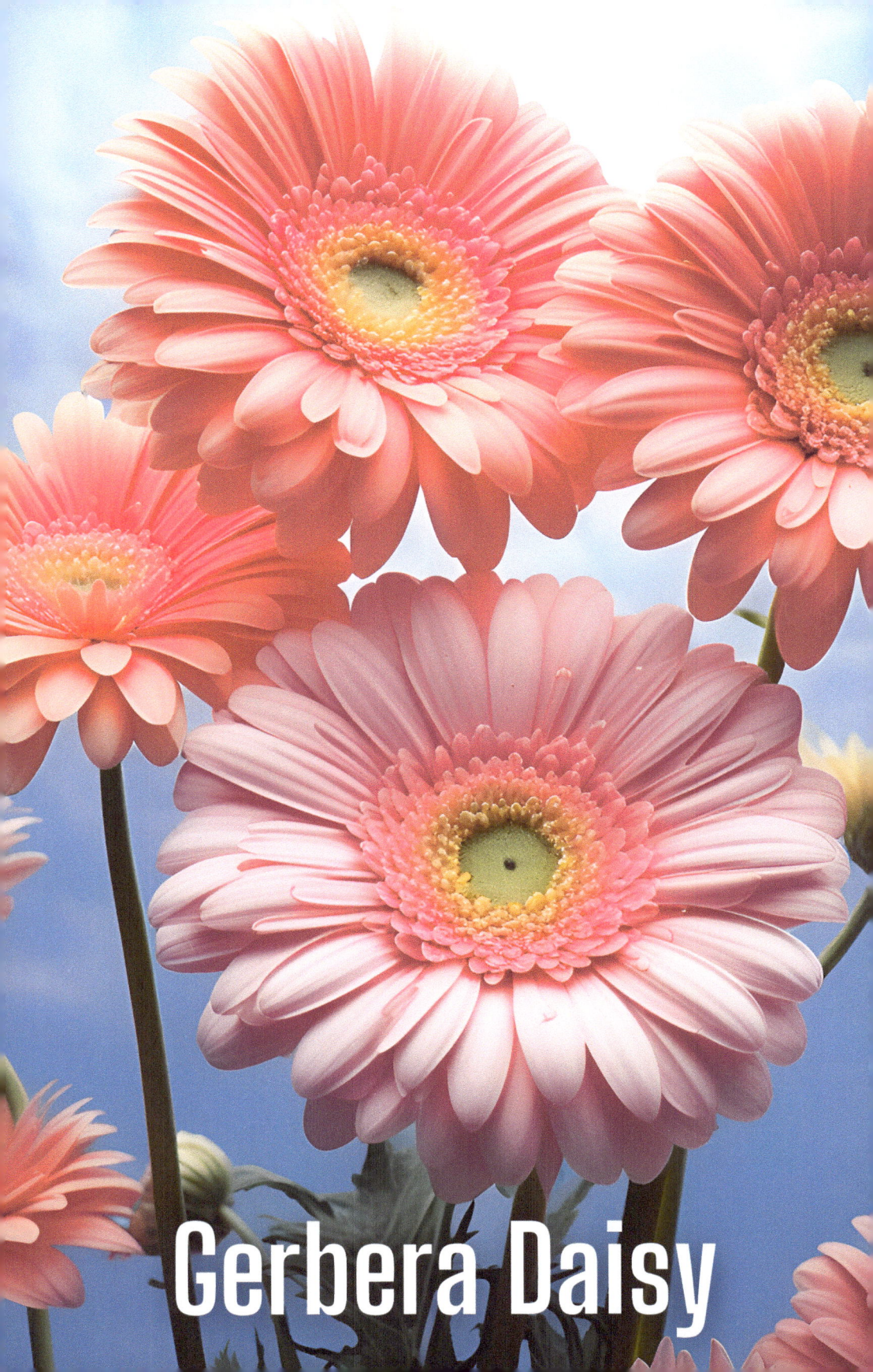

Gerbera Daisy

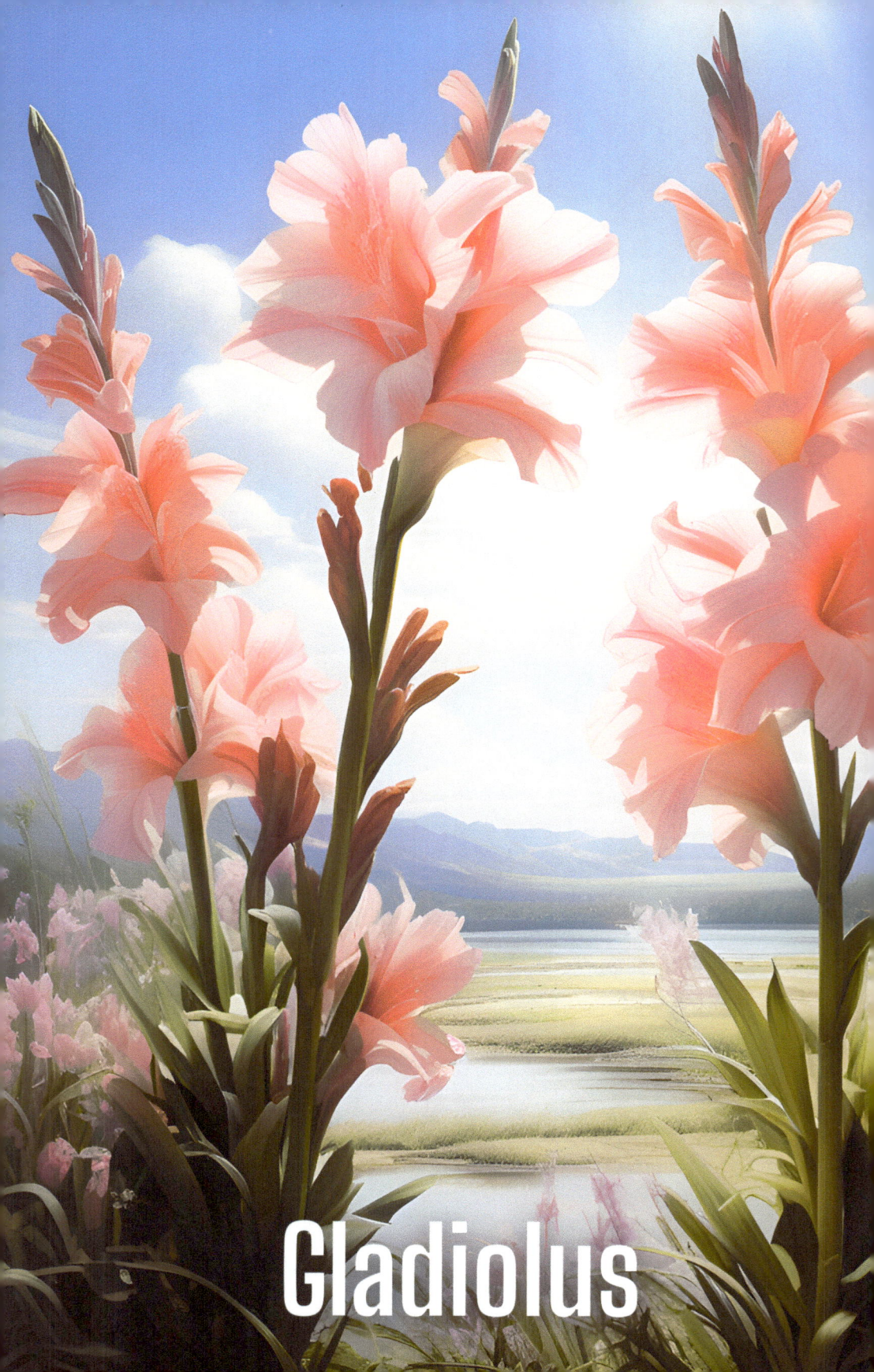

Gladiolus

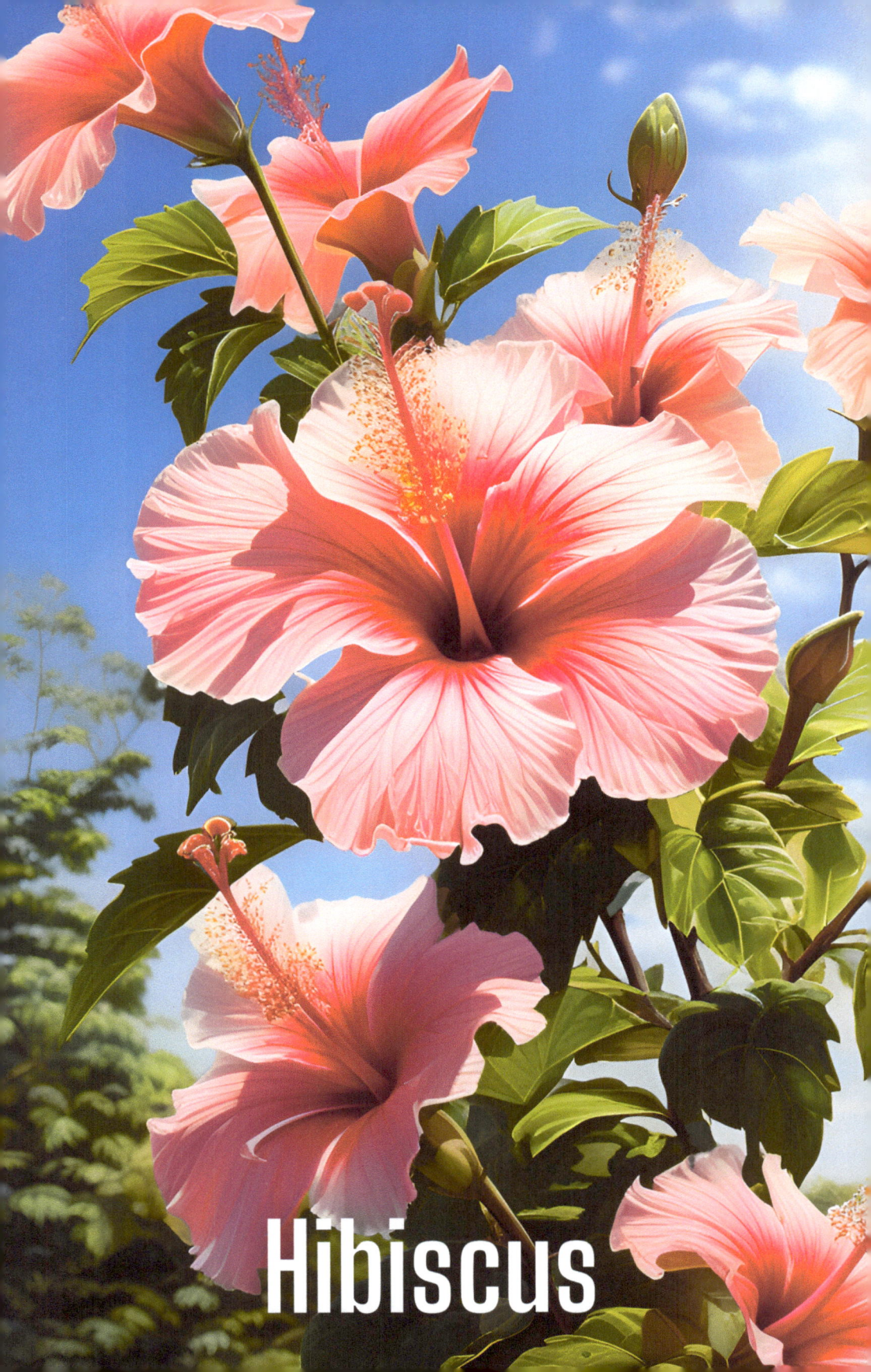

Hibiscus

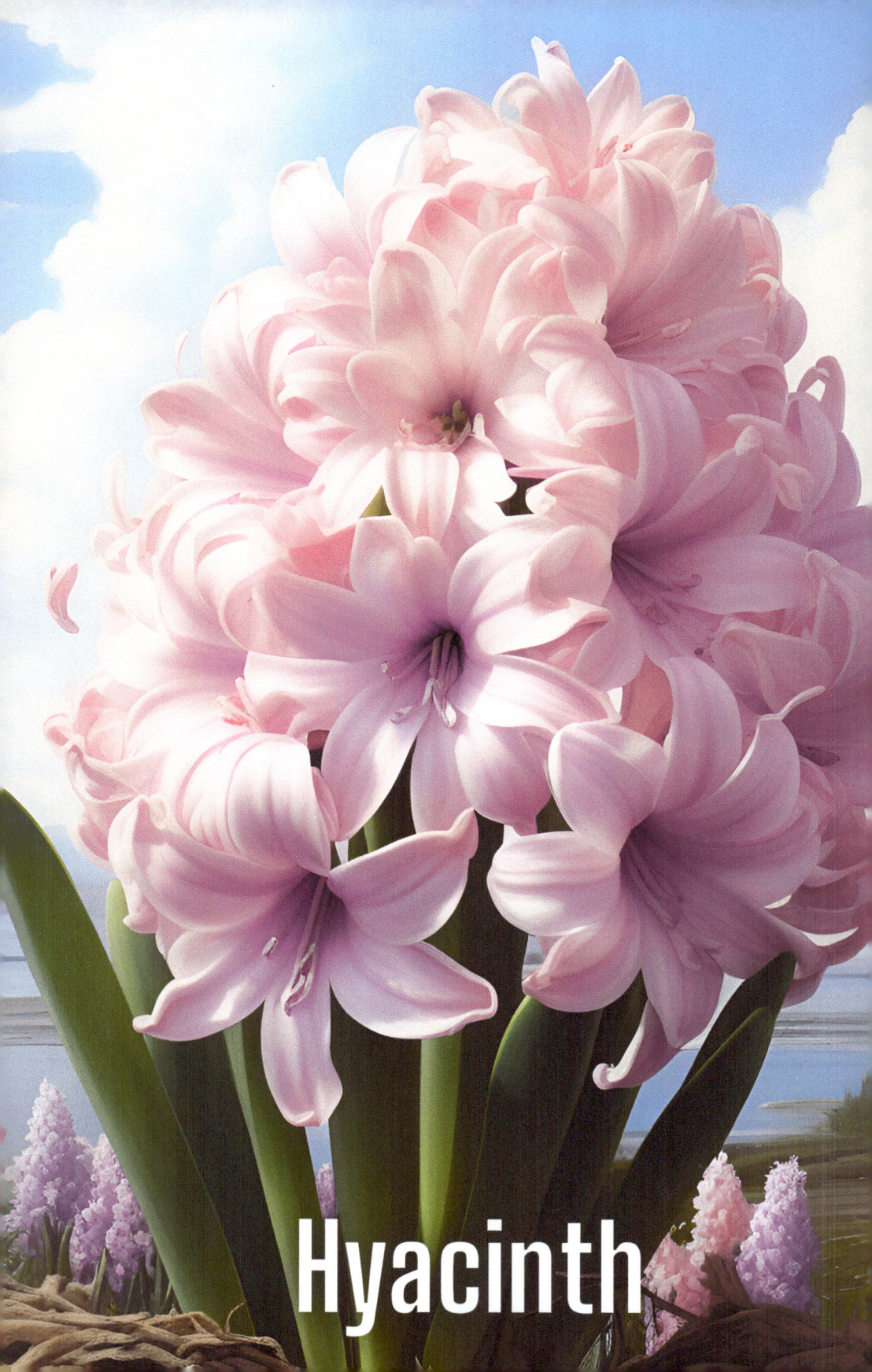

Hyacinth

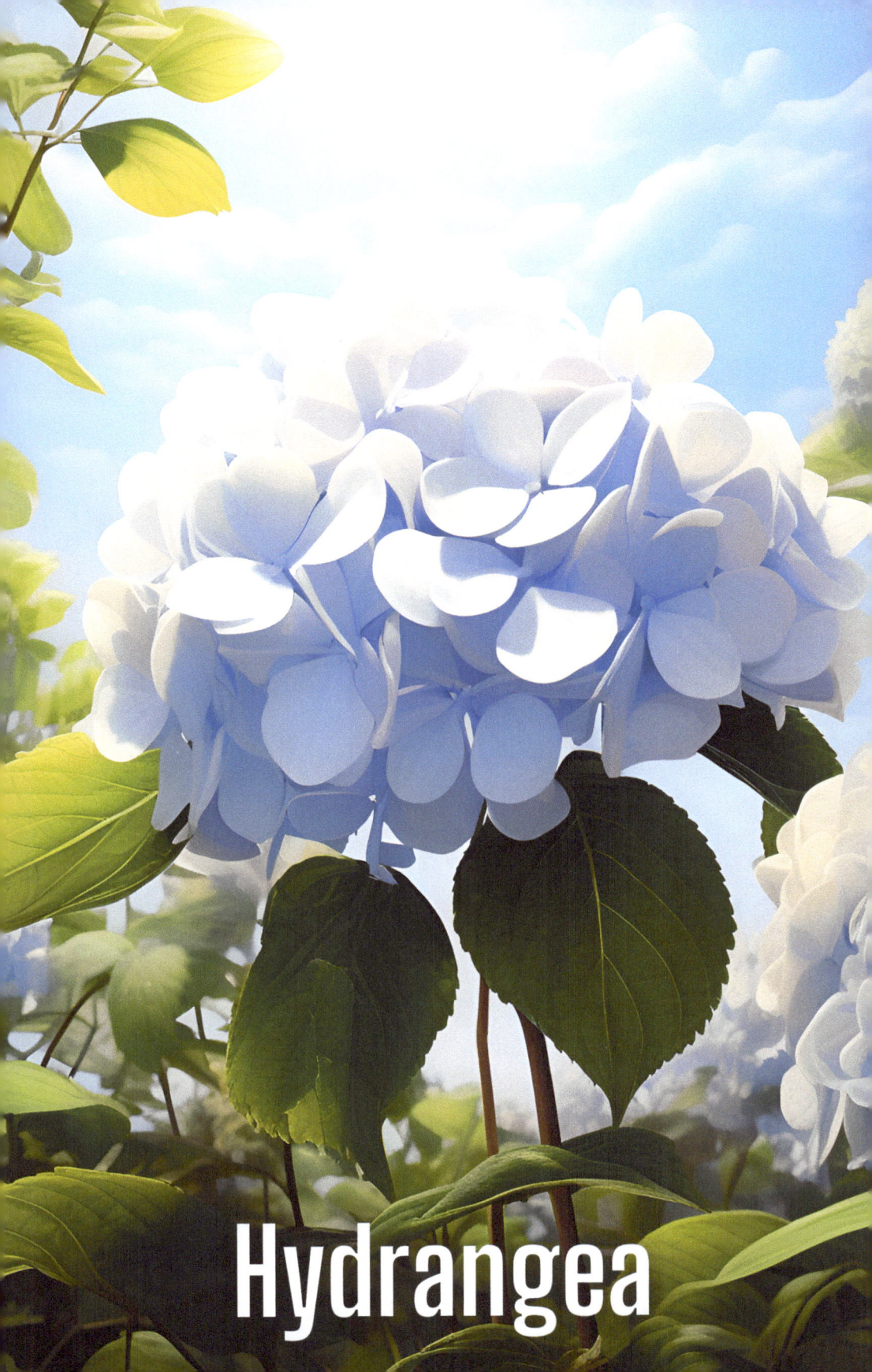

Hydrangea

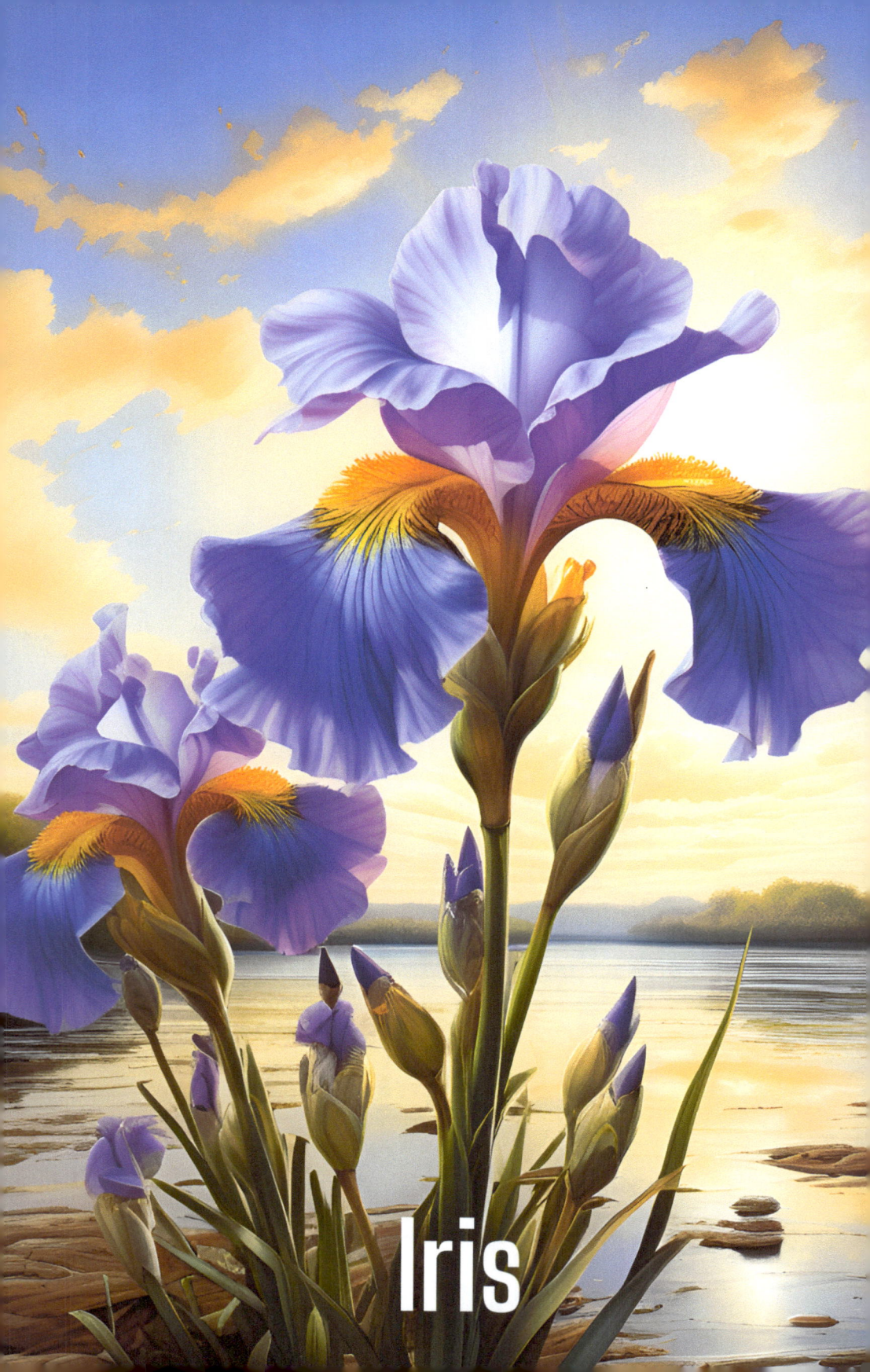

Iris

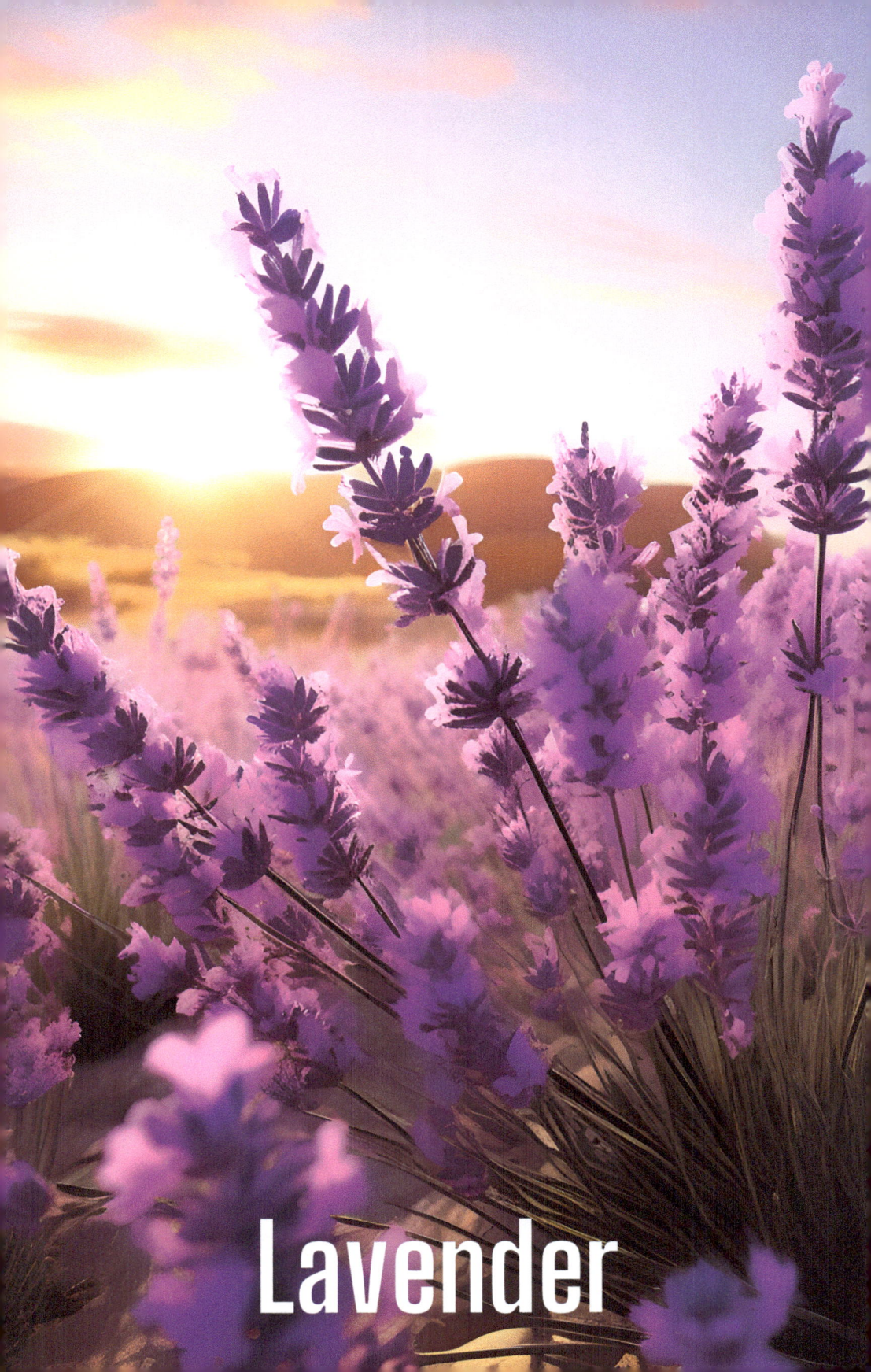

Lavender

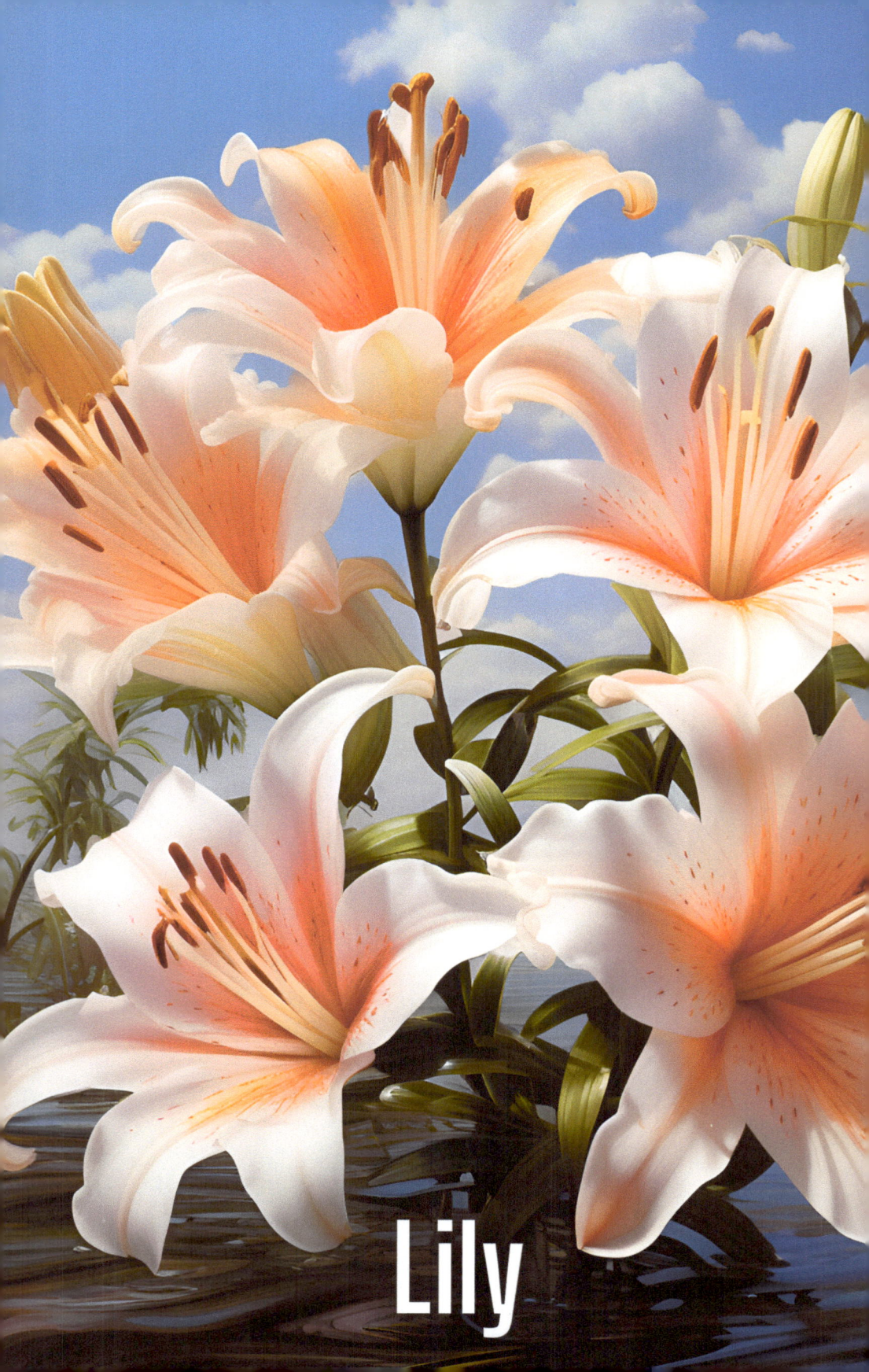

Lily

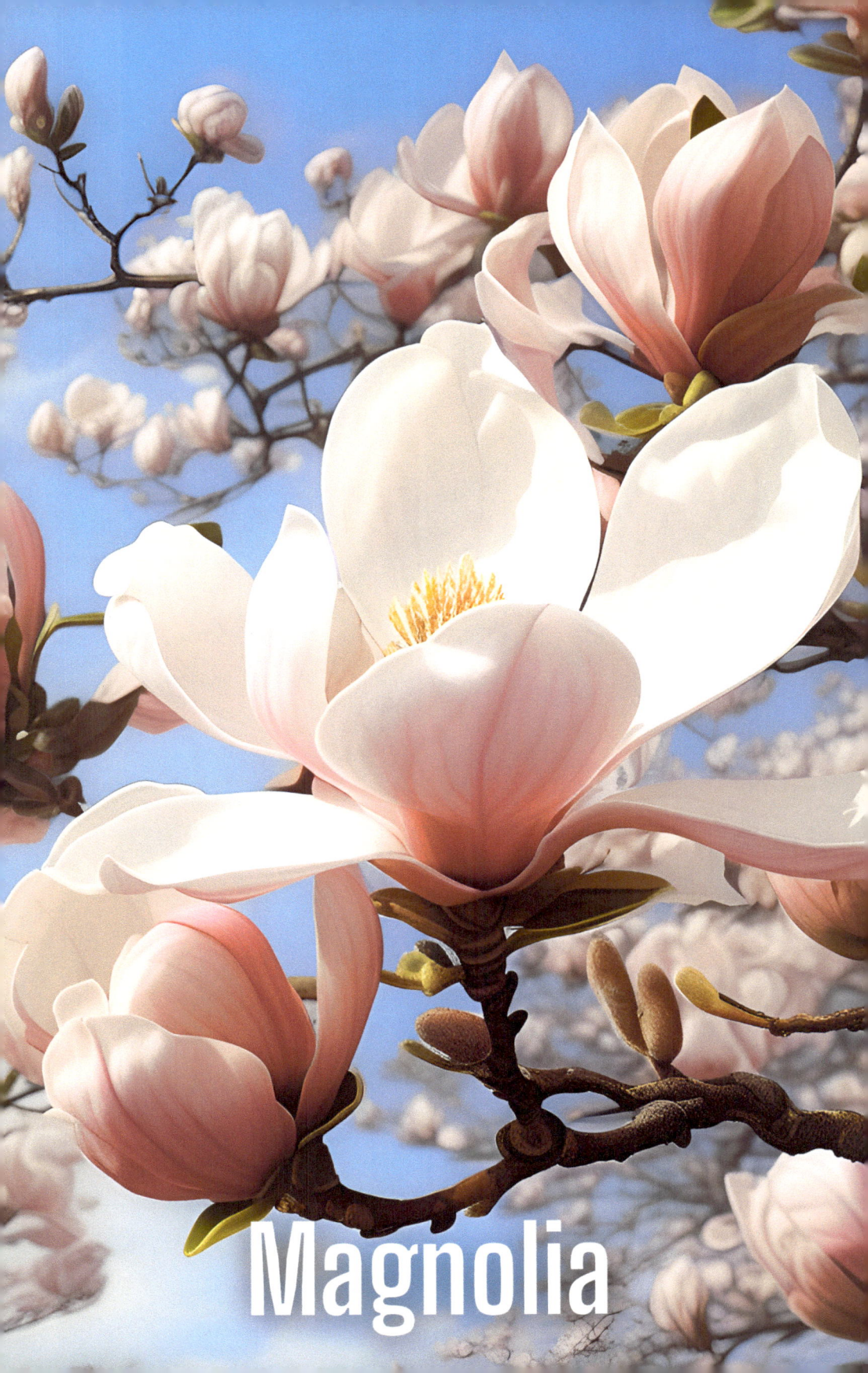

Magnolia

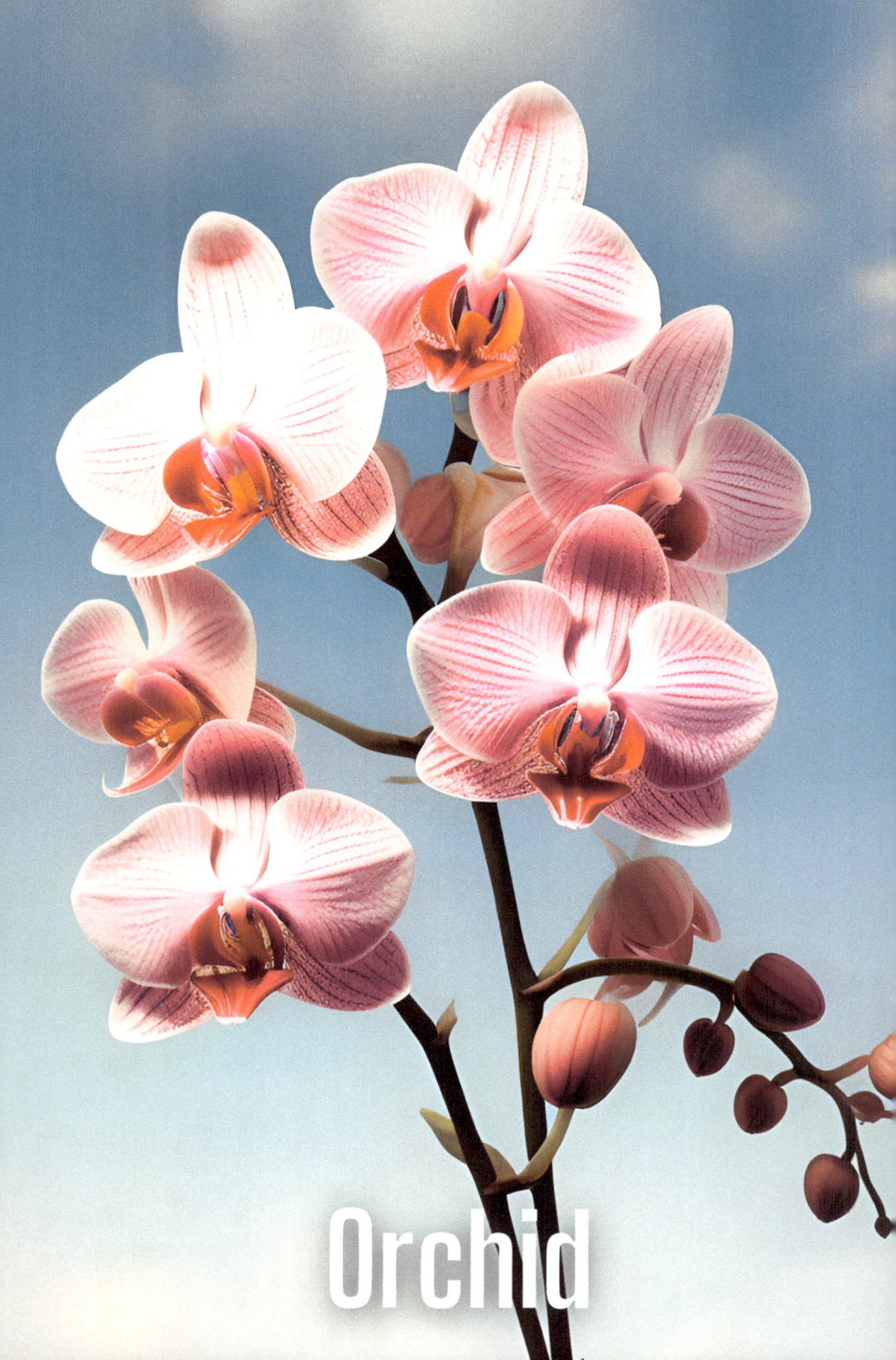

Orchid

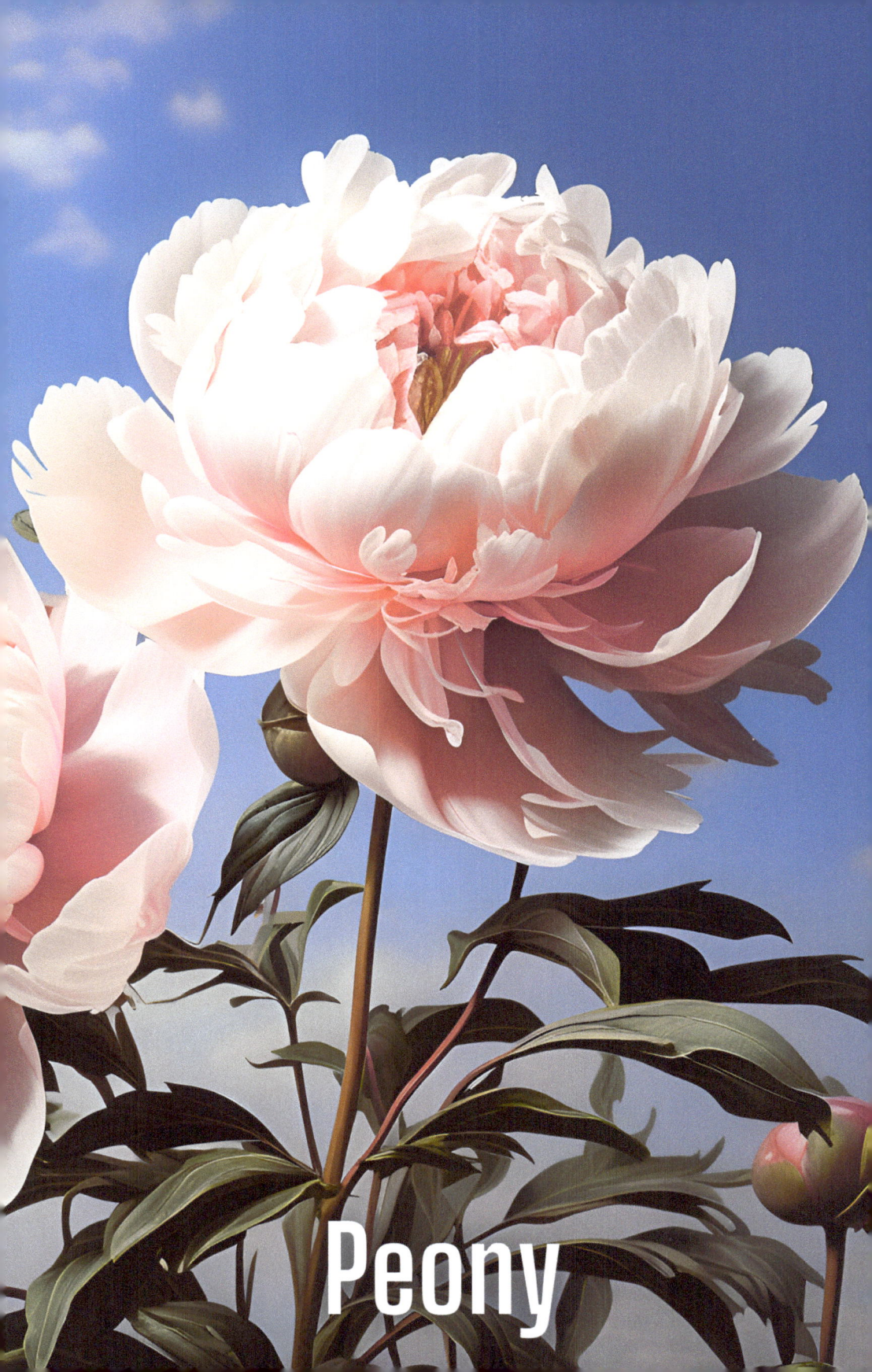

Peony

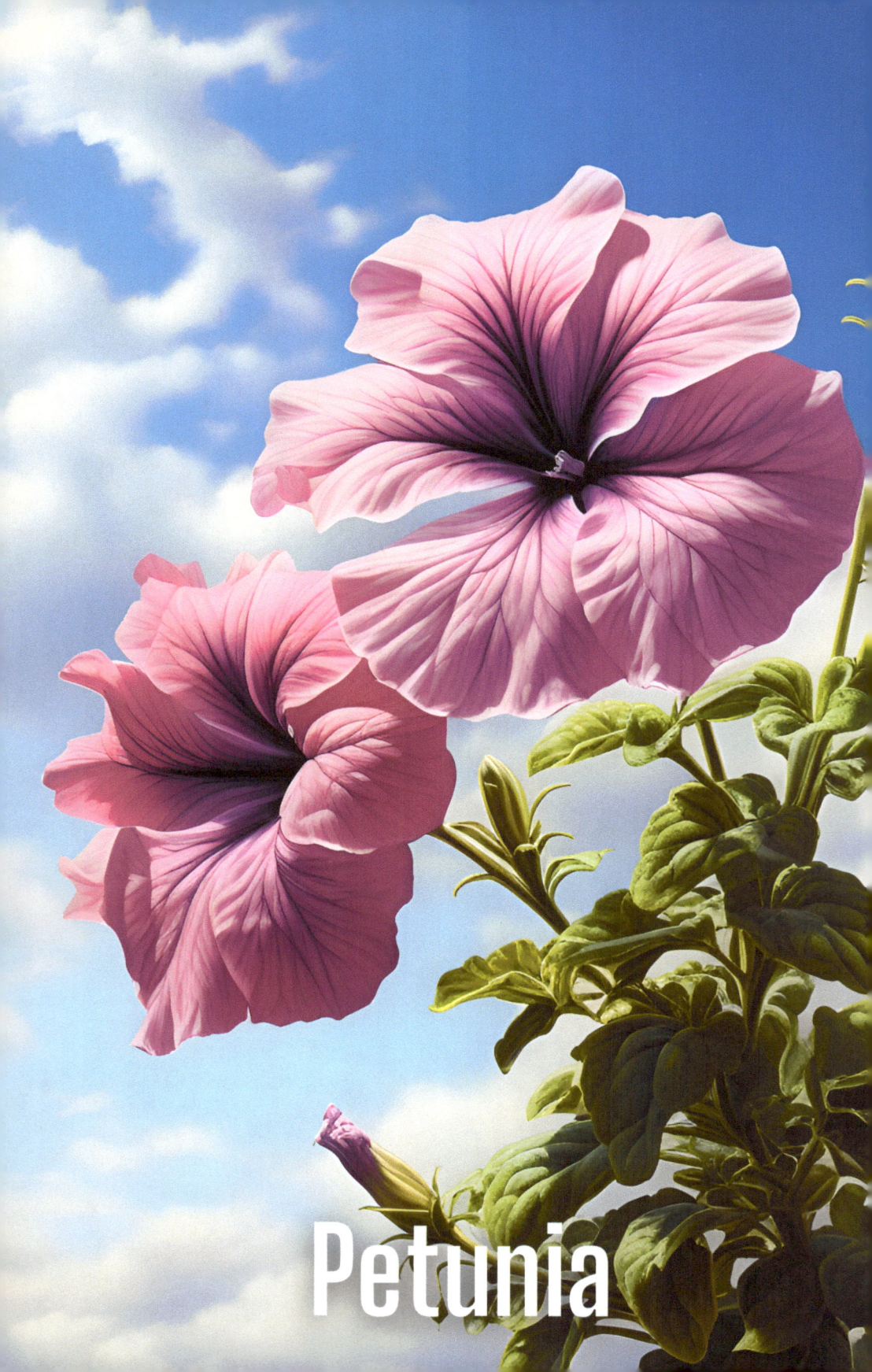

Petunia

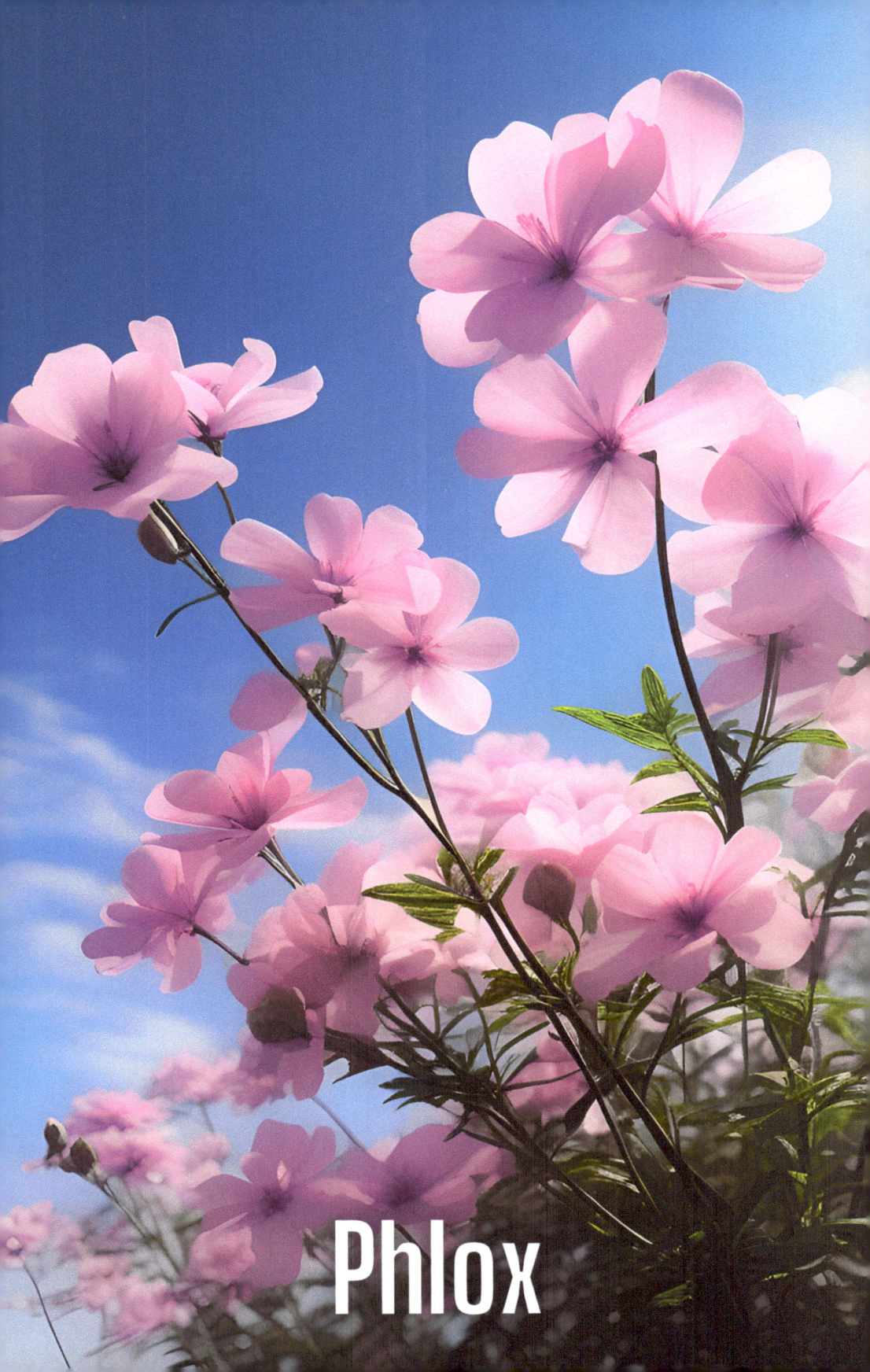

Phlox

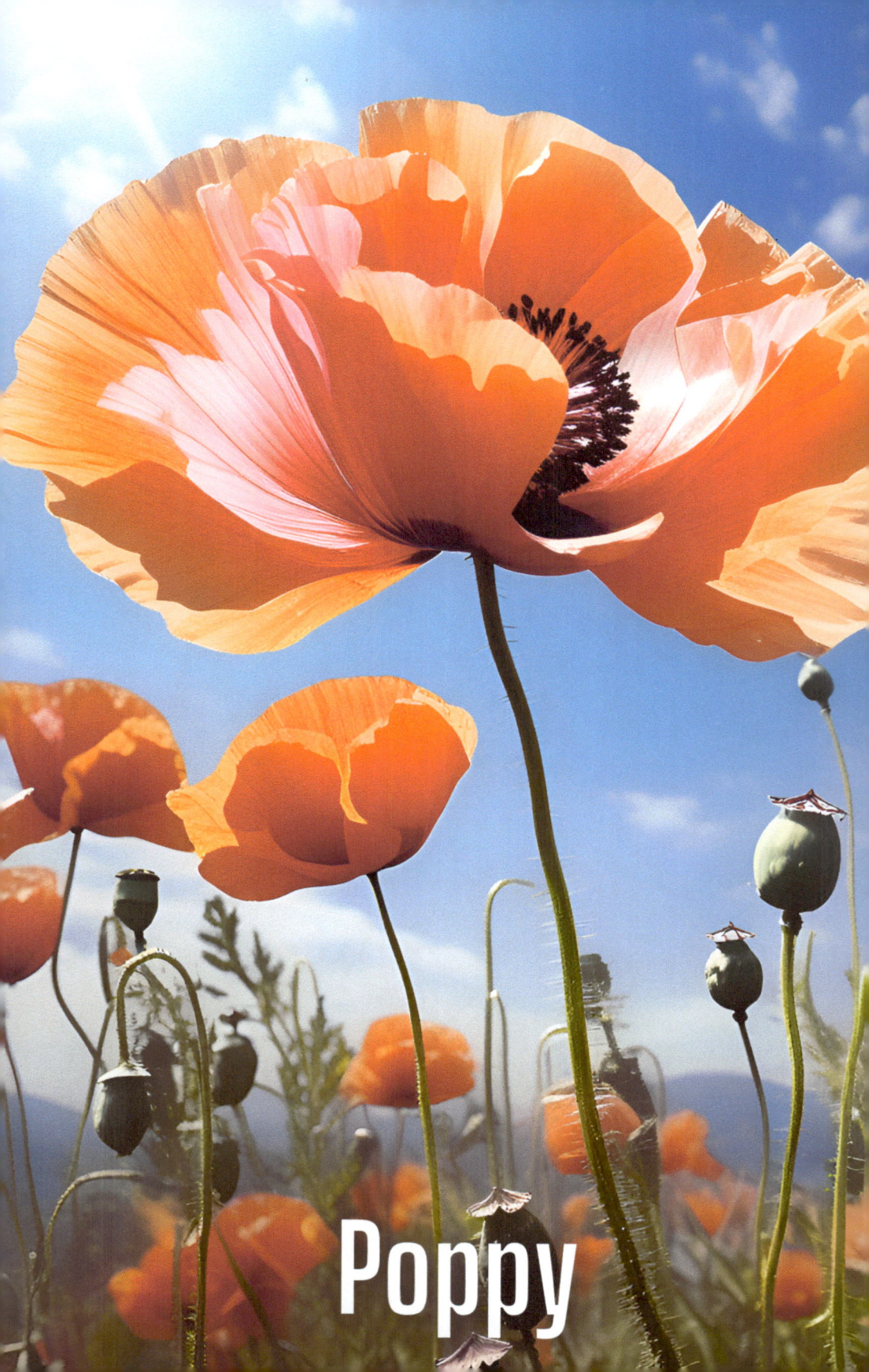

Poppy

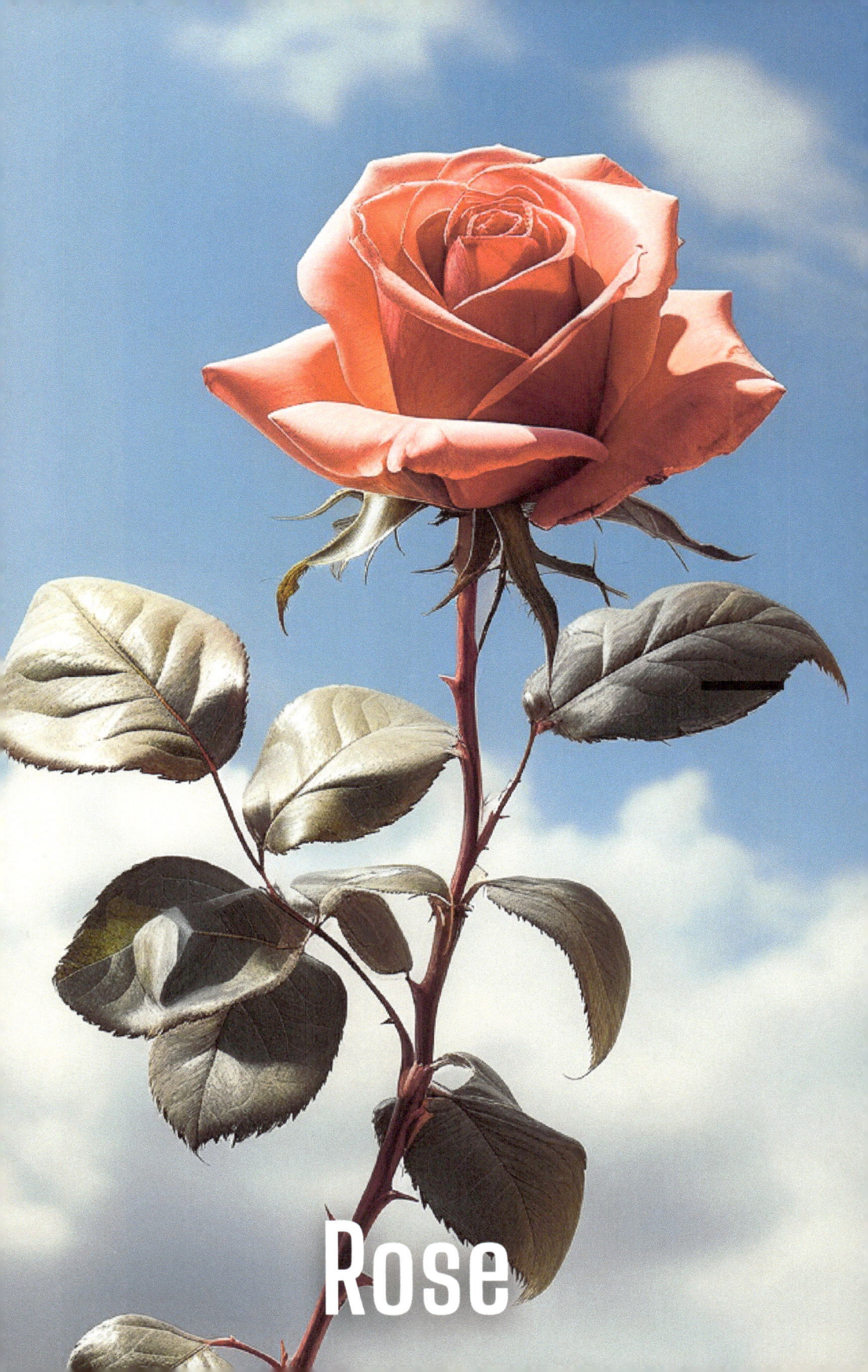

Rose

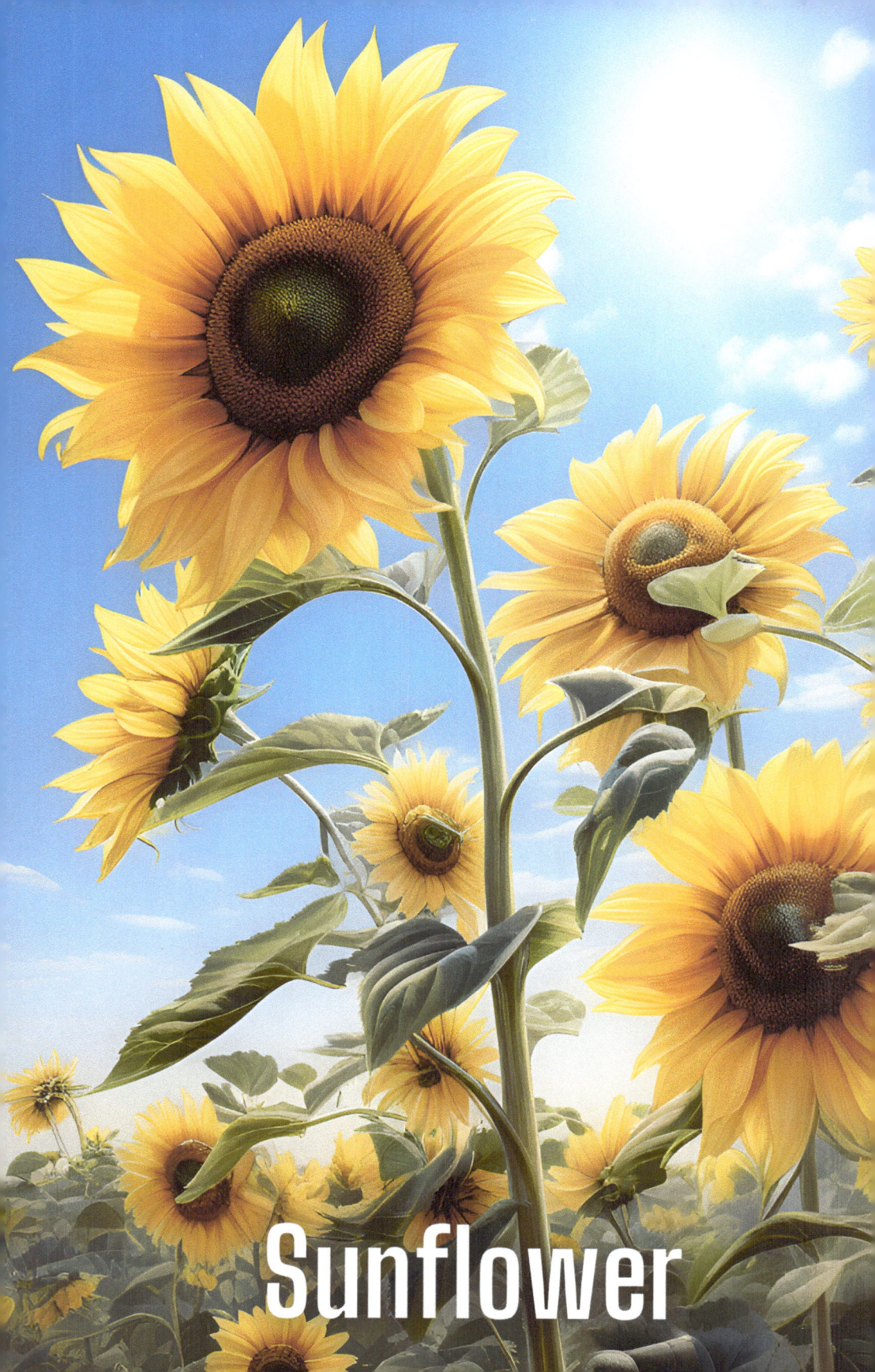

Sunflower

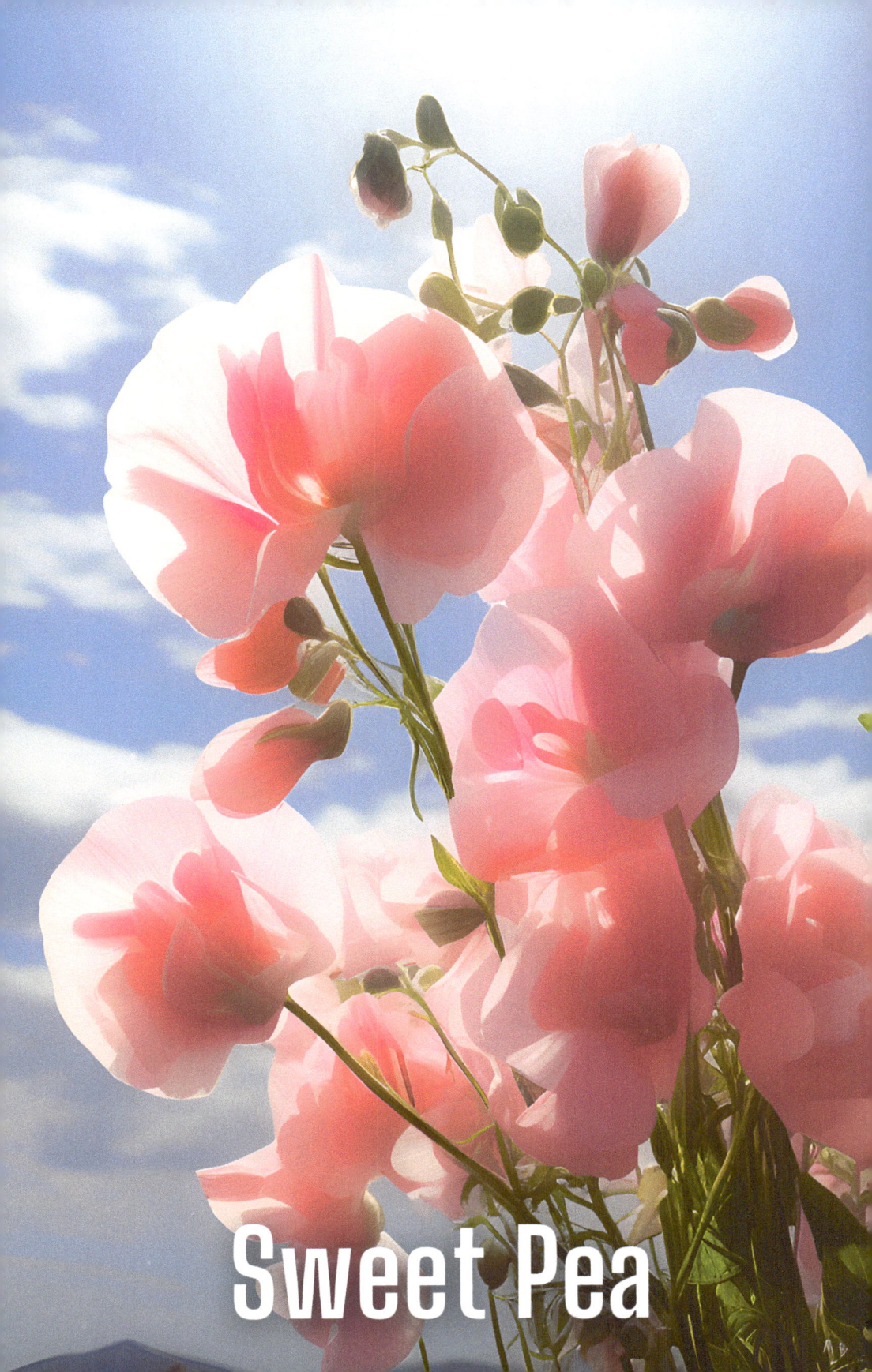

Sweet Pea

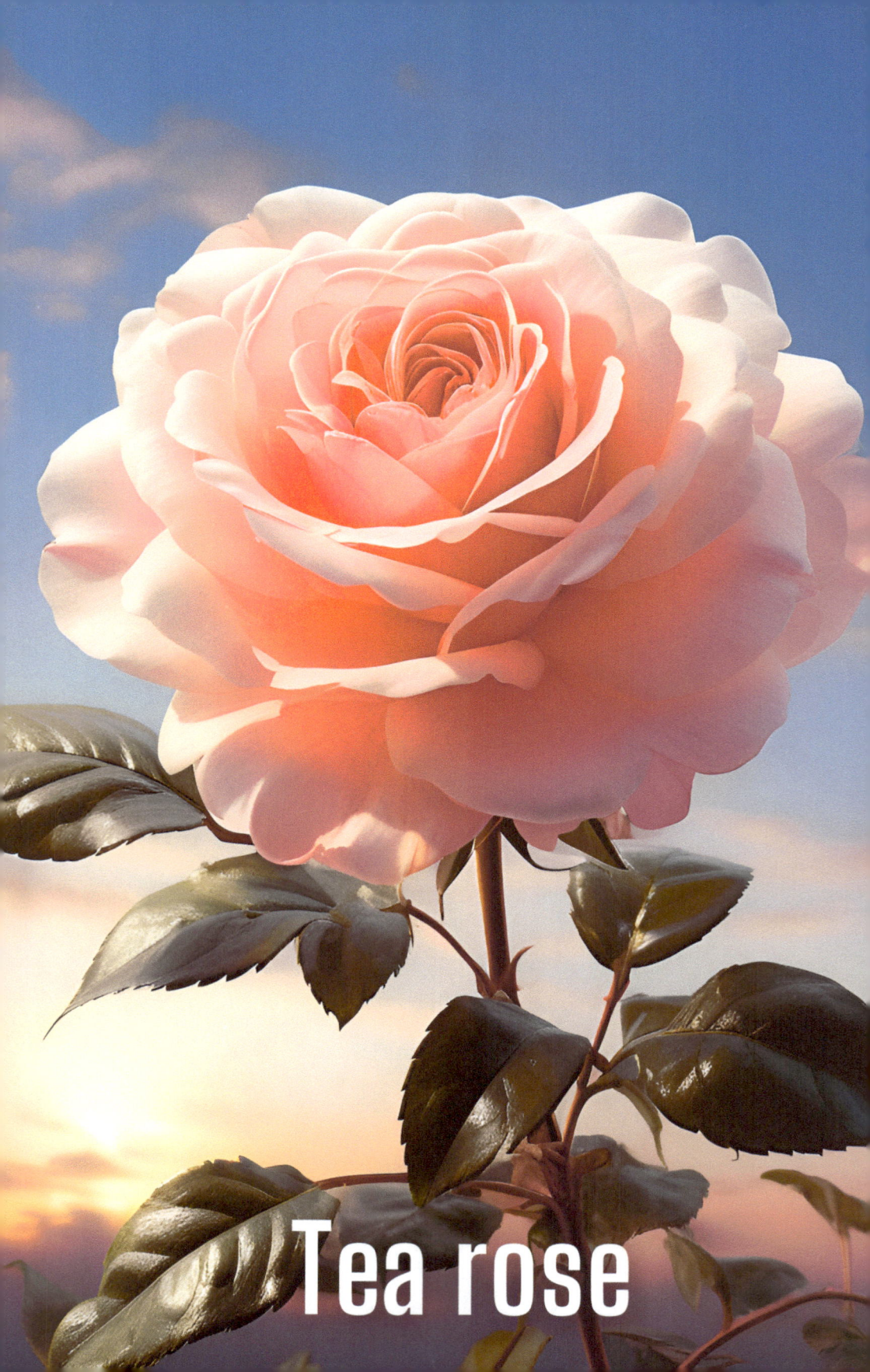

Tea rose

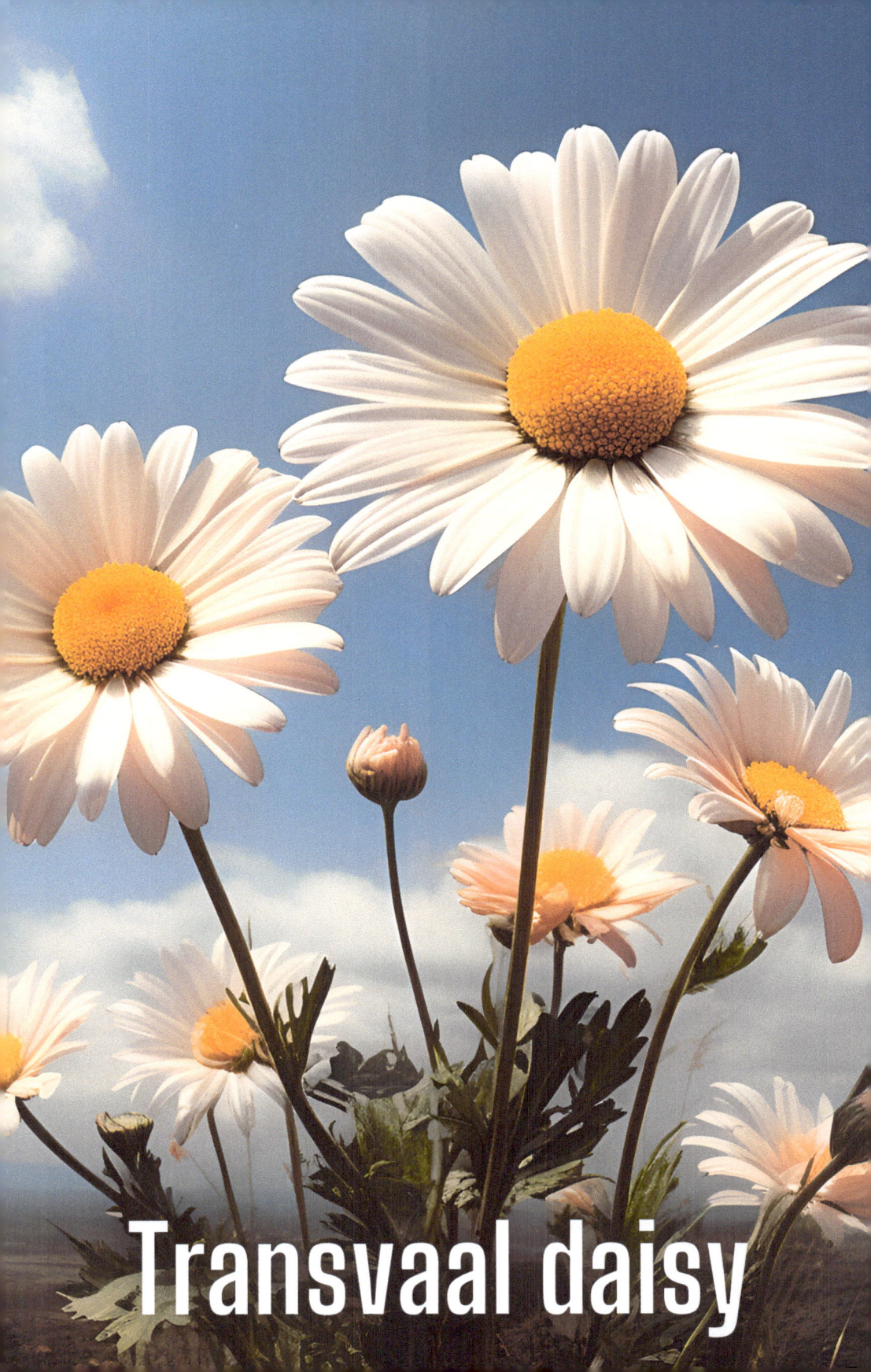

Transvaal daisy

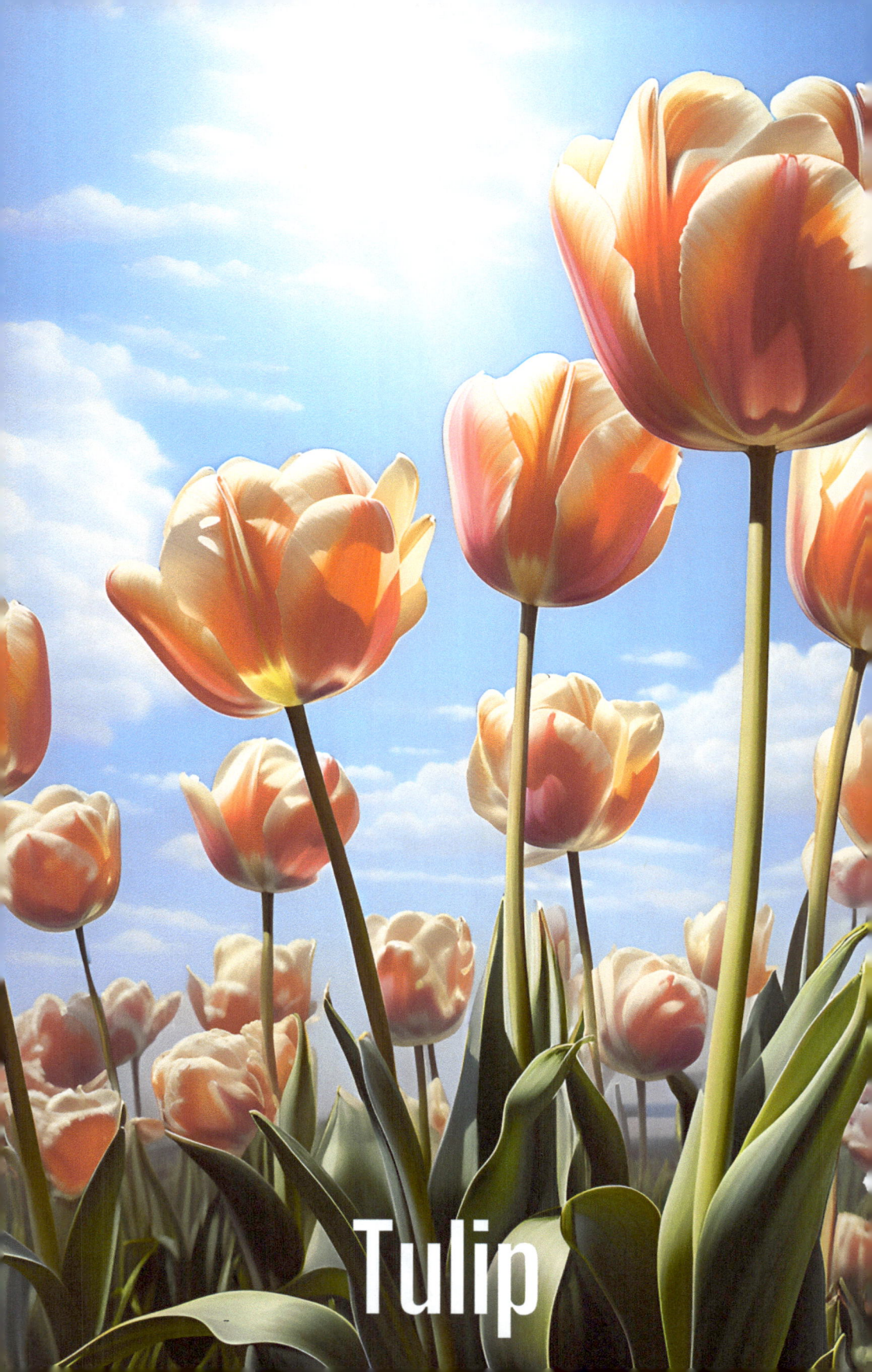

Tulip

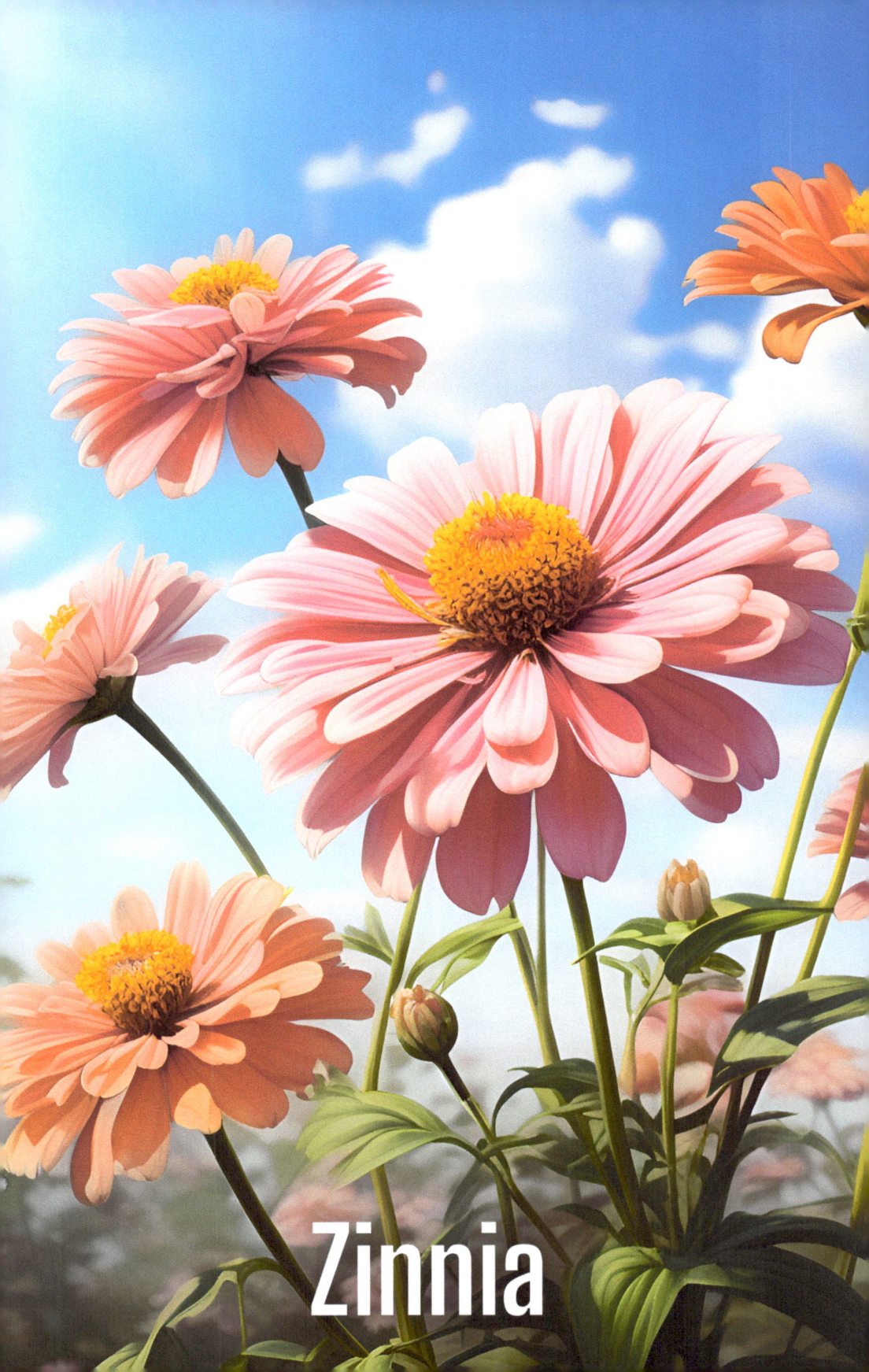

Zinnia

www.ingramcontent.com/pod-product-compliance
Lightning Source LLC
Chambersburg PA
CBHW050844290526
45792CB00002B/516